Cooking Light®
what to eat

ISBN-13: 978-0-8487-3320-9
ISBN-10: 0-8487-3320-7
Library of Congress Control Number: 2009937177
Printed in the United States of America
First Printing 2010

Be sure to check with your health-care provider
before making any changes in your diet.

Oxmoor House, Inc.

VP, Publishing Director: Jim Childs
Editorial Director: Susan Payne Dobbs
Brand Manager: Terri Laschober Robertson
Senior Editor: Heather Averett

Cooking Light® What to Eat

Editor: Rachel Quinlivan, R.D.
Project Editor: Diane Rose
Senior Designer: Emily Albright Parrish
Director, Test Kitchens: Elizabeth Tyler Austin
Assistant Director, Test Kitchens: Julie Christopher
Test Kitchens Professionals: Allison E. Cox, Julie Gunter,
    Kathleen Royal Phillips, Catherine Crowell Steele,
    Ashley T. Strickland
Photography Director: Jim Bathie
Senior Photo Stylist: Kay E. Clarke
Associate Photo Stylist: Katherine Eckert Coyne
Senior Production Manager: Greg A. Amason

Contributors

Copy Editor: Julie Gillis
Proofreader: Cathy Fowler
Indexer: Mary Ann Laurens
Interns: Ina Ables, Sarah Bellinger, Georgia Dodge,
    Perri K. Hubbard, Maggie McDaris, Allison Sperando
Test Kitchens Professional: Connie Nash
Photographer: Lee Harrelson
Photo Stylists: Missy Neville Crawford, Mindi Shapiro

Cooking Light®

Editor: Scott Mowbray
Creative Director: Carla Frank
Deputy Editor: Phillip Rhodes
Food Editor: Ann Taylor Pittman
Special Publications Editor: Mary Simpson Creel, M.S., R.D.
Nutrition Editor: Kathy Kitchens Downie, R.D.
Associate Food Editors: Timothy Q. Cebula, Julianna Grimes
Associate Editors: Cindy Hatcher, Brandy Rushing
Test Kitchens Director: Vanessa T. Pruett
Assistant Test Kitchens Director: Tiffany Vickers Davis
Senior Food Stylist: Kellie Gerber Kelley
Test Kitchens Professionals: SaBrina Bone, Deb Wise
Art Director: Fernande Bondarenko
Deputy Art Director: J. Shay McNamee
Photo Director: Kristen Schaefer
Senior Photographer: Randy Mayor
Senior Photo Stylist: Cindy Barr
Photo Stylist: Leigh Ann Ross
Copy Chief: Maria Parker Hopkins
Assistant Copy Chief: Susan Roberts
Research Editor: Michelle Gibson Daniels
Editorial Production Director: Liz Rhoades
Production Editor: Hazel R. Eddins
CookingLight.com Editor: Allison Long Lowery
Art/Production Assistant: Josh Rutledge
Administrative Coordinator: Carol D. Johnson

To order additional publications,
call 1–800–765–6400 or 1-800-491-0551.

For more books to enrich your life,
visit **oxmoorhouse.com**

To search, savor, and share thousands of recipes,
visit **myrecipes.com**

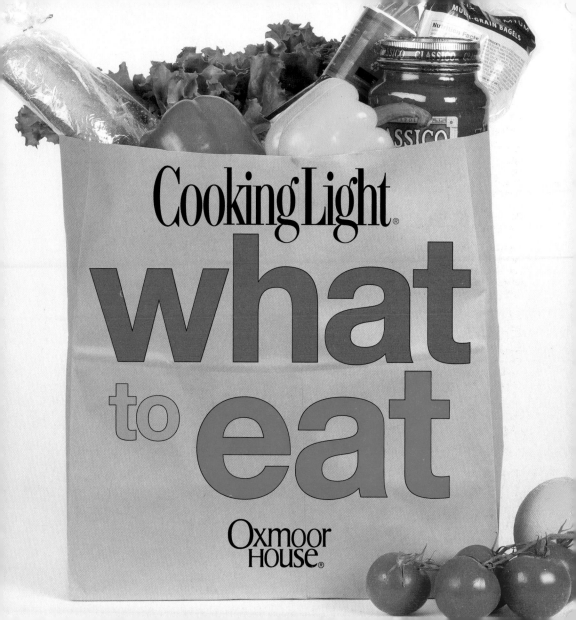

Cooking Light®
what
to eat

Oxmoor House®

contents

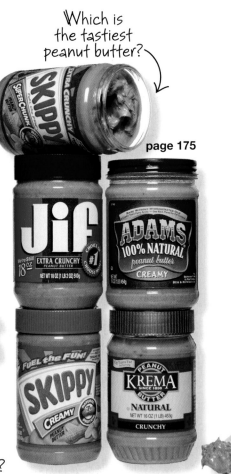

Which is the tastiest peanut butter?

page 175

What's the deal with saturated fats?

page 22

page 233

How much is a serving of ice cream?

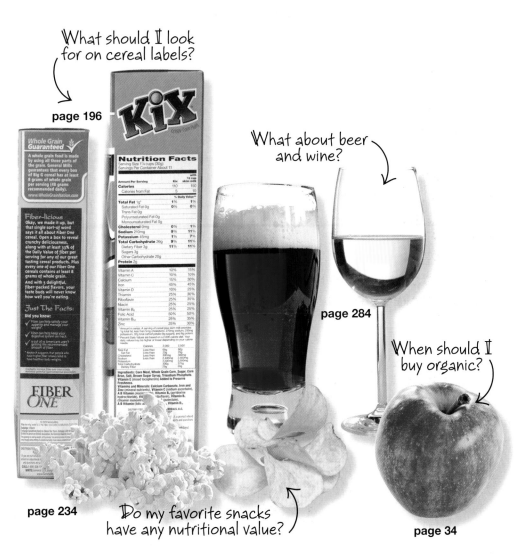

What should I look for on cereal labels?

page 196

What about beer and wine?

page 284

When should I buy organic?

page 34

page 234

Do my favorite snacks have any nutritional value?

what to eat?

With so many products available in today's grocery stores, that question is often a complicated one for many people who are trying to find foods that fit their nutritional goals. With low-sugar, no-sugar, low-carb, all-natural, organic, and all the other health claims attached to food packages and nutrition labels, healthy eating can be stressful—but it shouldn't be.

That's where this book comes in. It isn't filled with a list of specific brands of products that may be outdated in a week (although we do provide some of our favorite picks that we use regularly). Instead, we've distilled healthy eating into a set of straightforward guidelines that take you aisle by aisle through the grocery store.

We teach you what to look for on the package and the nutrition label—for any product—to help you make the healthiest choice from the options in front of you. We give you the facts. They're the very same ones we use when we're standing in the bread aisle (or the canned food aisle or the meat section or the freezer section) choosing from the hundreds of options. We want to help you eat healthy and get the most nutritional bang for your grocery store dollar. Here's how.

—Scott Mowbray, Editor

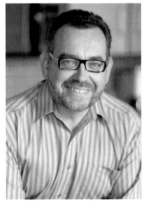

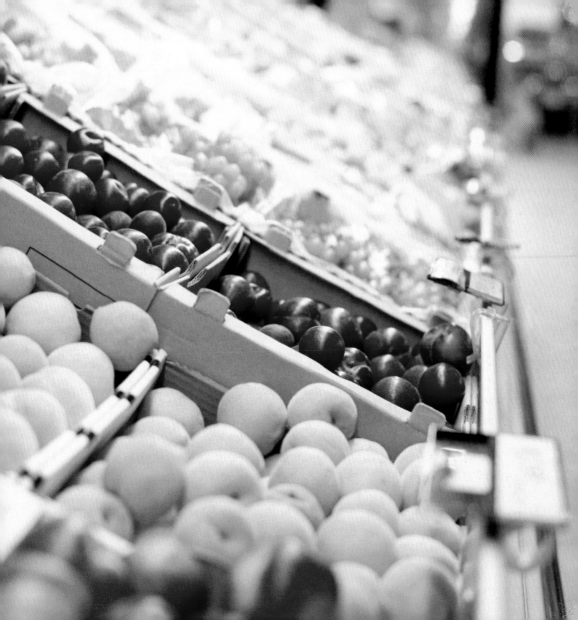

our grocery
store guide

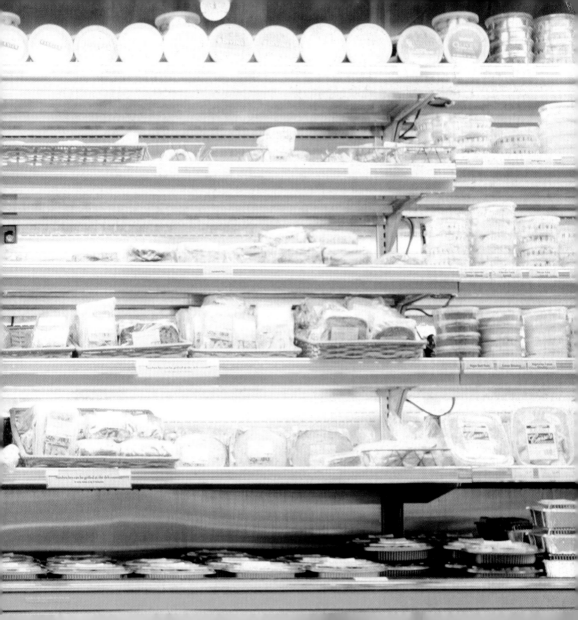

our guide to the <mark>healthiest</mark> shopping

Healthy eating begins in the grocery store. Here are the basic tips for getting started—they'll help your health and your budget.

1. Base meals on items from the grocery store perimeter.

Shopping along the outside edges of the grocery store is the easiest way to amp up the nutritional quality of what you eat. That's because the perimeter is where a majority of stores feature inherently healthy foods—fresh fruits and vegetables, fish, meats, poultry, and dairy products. You'll also want to shop the aisles containing 100% whole-grain breads and pastas and whole grains such as oatmeal, barley, and quinoa.

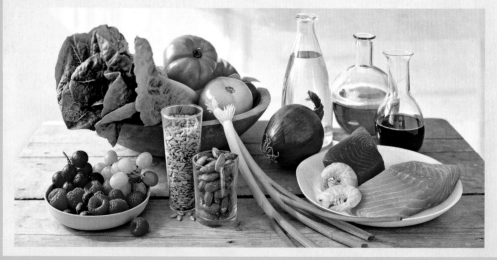

2. Compare apples to apples (and chicken to chicken).

Compare the prices of similar items. Make sure you're comparing pound per pound and serving per serving. Say you're considering a $7.50 package of skinless, boneless chicken breasts versus a $3.50 whole chicken. That $7.50 package with two chicken breasts is just over a pound and will feed two to three people, while the whole chicken is more than three pounds and will feed four, as well as make homemade chicken stock and soup.

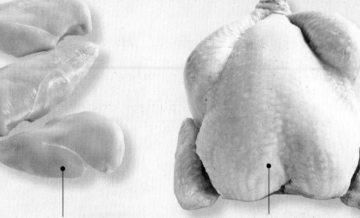

skinless, boneless chicken breasts: $5.49 per pound

whole chicken: $1.28 per pound

3. Look high and low.

Prime product placement in grocery stores goes for a premium price—vendors sometimes pay retailers thousands of dollars for placement at middle and eye-level shelves. These products may be some of the healthiest and most affordable ones, but make sure you also check the upper and lower shelves for good (and nutritious) deals.

our guide to the healthiest shopping, continued

4. Buy in bulk.

Buying in bulk the foods you eat often can save you money. Steel-cut oats bought from the bulk bin, for instance, are $0.89 per pound, while a tin runs $3.35 a pound. Lentils, beans, and chickpeas are also great bulk savers, as well as large bags of rice. However, not all foods are cheaper in bulk, so you'll need to do your homework to be sure. See page 11 for information about comparing the prices of similar items.

5. Buy seasonally.

Seasonal produce offers more than just freshness and delicious taste—it also saves money. Cucumbers, for example, are generally bargains in season. But out of season, they have to travel from afar and can cost several dollars per pound. Stay attuned to the seasons so you can buy the fruits and veggies that are the most economical and freshest.

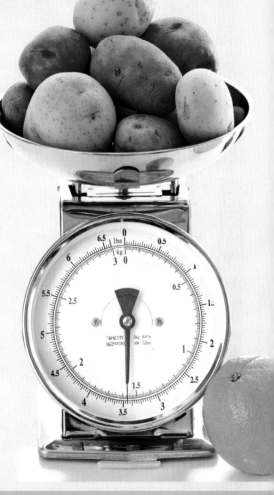

6. Read the Nutrition Facts labels and the ingredient lists.

Since 1994, the Food and Drug Administration has required products to carry Nutrition Facts labels that list the amount of calories, calories from fat, total and saturated fat, protein, carbohydrates, fiber, sugar, cholesterol, sodium, vitamins A and C, calcium, and iron per serving. The most recent addition is trans fat (added in 2006). Many companies have also voluntarily included additional information, such as levels of potassium and mono- and polyunsaturated fats. Read the labels: Studies show those who read Nutrition Facts labels are more likely to eat less foods high in saturated fat than those who don't.

All products are required to list the ingredients that are used to make that product. This is especially beneficial when determining if a product contains unhealthy trans fats. See page 22 for more information about trans fats.

our guide to the healthiest shopping, continued

7. **Make sure you understand what the health claims really mean.**

You'll find a variety of health claims—trans fat free, made with whole grains, all natural—splashed across the packages of a variety of products, but those healthy-sounding phrases don't always tell the whole story. For example, a package may say "trans fat free," but, by law, a product can claim to be trans fat free if it has less than 0.5 grams of trans fat *per serving*. The real way to see if the product is truly free of trans fats is to check the ingredient list to be sure you don't see the words "partially hydrogenated oil." If you do, the product has trans fats, despite what the label claims. We've included tips throughout this book to help you understand package labels.

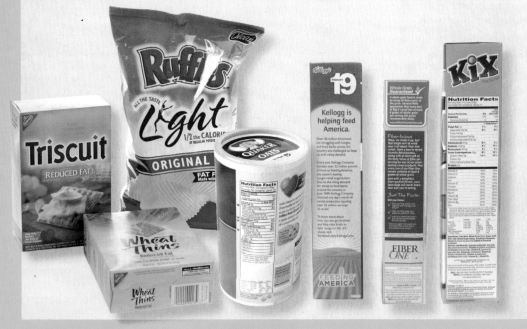

8. Store brands can be just as good as brand names.

Store-brand products can be tasty and nutritious, and they can help keep your grocery bill in check. Store brands can cost a fraction of the price of brand names—around 25% less. The difference in price is usually not from differences in what goes into the food but rather the marketing and promotion costs that come with building a brand into a household favorite.

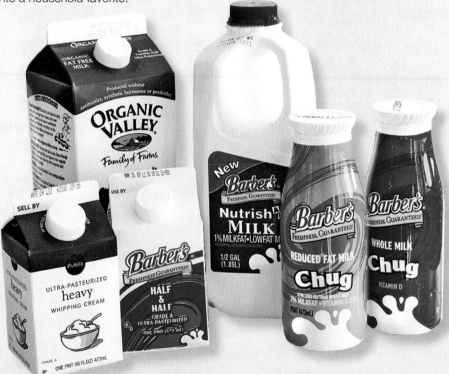

our guide to the healthiest shopping, continued

9. Weigh the cost of convenience foods.

With convenience comes a heftier price tag. For example, whole broccoli runs $1.69 per pound, while a bag of precut broccoli florets comes in at $3.36 per pound. In cases such as these, you might want to consider if the extra cost is really worth the time saved by having someone else cut up your broccoli for you.

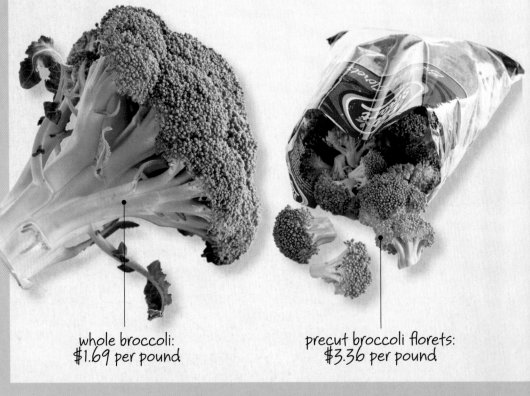

whole broccoli:
$1.69 per pound

precut broccoli florets:
$3.36 per pound

10. Shop for bargains.

Check your local grocery store's weekly circular, or look for specials at the store to plan meals around the items that are on sale. When there's a sale on items you use regularly, take advantage and buy extra. "Buy-one, get-one-free" deals, in particular, can help your bottom line.

our guide to the healthiest eating

Healthy eating doesn't have to be a mystery. Follow these guidelines to help you get started.

1. Variety is the spice of life.

Time and again, research points to eating a variety of foods for optimal health—wonderful news for anyone who enjoys eating. Choose fruits and vegetables in all the colors of the rainbow, and eat lots of them (see page 30 for the United States Department of Agriculture's recommendations). Reach for whole grains, beans, legumes, and a wide range of lean protein.

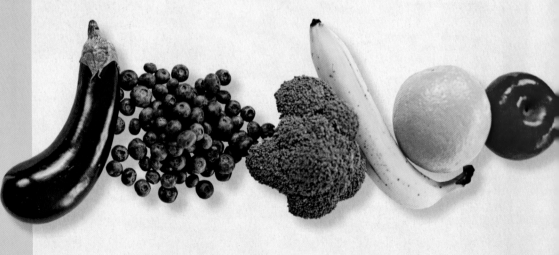

2. Slash sodium.

For most people, the more sodium you consume, the higher your blood pressure will be. And as blood pressure jumps, so does the risk for heart disease and stroke. The American Heart Association and the USDA's Dietary Guidelines for Americans suggest limiting sodium to less than 2,300 milligrams a day (the amount in one teaspoon of salt) for healthy adults and 1,500 milligrams per day for those who are salt sensitive—typically individuals who have high blood pressure, are 40 years of age or older, or who are African-American. More than two-thirds of the adult population falls into one or more of these categories.

daily sodium limit for adults: scant 1 teaspoon salt = 2,300mg sodium

daily sodium the average American consumes: heaping 1½ teaspoons salt = 4,000mg sodium

3. Choose healthy fats.

Research has shown that it's the *type* of fat you eat, and not so much the amount, that has the biggest effect on health. Fats are indispensable. They deliver essential fatty acids that the body cannot manufacture, such as omega-3s, which bolster heart health. Also, certain vitamins are fat-soluble, meaning they are digested and absorbed or transported in the body with fat. (These include vitamins A, D, E, and K.) However, fats are high in calories, so you should enjoy them in moderation. The good-for-you fats are those that are unsaturated—monounsaturated and polyunsaturated—and the unhealthy ones include saturated fat and trans fats. The key is striking a balance between them. The following pages contain the information you need to know about each.

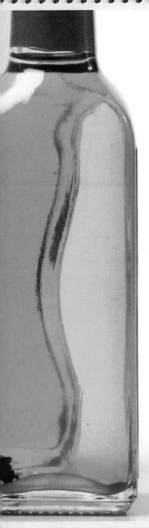

monounsaturated fats

These plant-based fats are liquid at room temperature and can help lower cholesterol when used in place of saturated fat in the diet.

Sources: Canola, olive, and peanut oils, as well as peanuts, pecans, and avocados.

polyunsaturated fats

These plant- and fish-derived fats can lower cholesterol when they replace saturated fat in the diet. Fatty fish like salmon and tuna contain their own special variety of polyunsaturated fats called omega-3 fatty acids, which appear to keep the heart healthy, even when consumed in small amounts. Certain nuts, oils, and greens offer another type of omega-3 fats. Eating plant sources of these omega-3 fats, such as flaxseed and walnuts, likely helps keep bones strong.

Sources: Vegetable oils like safflower, sunflower, soybean, corn, and sesame oils. Sunflower seeds; soybeans; fatty fish like tuna, mackerel, and salmon; and most nuts are also rich in these fats.

our guide to the healthiest eating, continued

trans fats

Produced when liquid oils are processed into solid shortenings, trans fats raise "bad" LDL cholesterol and lower "good" HDL cholesterol. Some meat and dairy products, such as beef, lamb, and butterfat, contain naturally occurring trans fats. It's unclear whether these natural trans fats have the same negative effects as manufactured trans fats. The American Heart Association recommends limiting the amount of trans fat you eat to less than 1% of your total daily calories—about 2 grams for the average person on a 2,000-calorie-a-day diet. Given the amount of naturally occurring trans fats most people likely eat every day, there's not much room, if any, for manufactured trans fats. (See page 14 for more information about trans-fats labeling.)

Sources: Foods that contain partially hydrogenated oils, which are found primarily in processed food, such as french fries, doughnuts, pastries, pie crusts, biscuits, pizza dough, crackers, cookies, stick margarines, and shortenings.

saturated fats

Concentrated mostly in animal products, these fats are solid at room temperature. They raise harmful LDL cholesterol and increase the risk for heart disease. The American Heart Association advises limiting saturated fats to less than 7% of total calories—about 15 grams for the average person on a 2,000-calorie-a-day diet.

Sources: Beef, lamb, pork, bacon, cheese, full-fat yogurt, butter, whole milk, and snack chips and bakery items made with tropical oils like coconut, palm, and palm kernel.

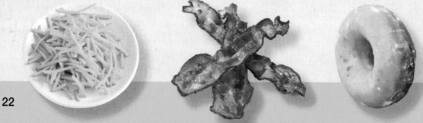

4. Be aware of portion sizes.

The secret of healthy eating is this: Once you know what makes up a healthy diet, you still need to be aware of *how much* of those components to eat. Some tips: Use smaller plates, cups, and serving utensils—you'll serve (and eat) smaller portions. You may also want to measure food with measuring cups or weigh it using a food scale. Recognizing what a reasonable portion looks like without measuring or weighing will eventually become automatic, but measuring and weighing food to start with can help you reach that point. We provide serving-size guidelines in each chapter to help you spot a proper portion.

our guide to the healthiest eating, continued

5. Go for whole grains.

Research has shown that eating just 2½ servings of whole grains per day is enough to lower your risk for heart disease. (One serving equals a slice of 100% whole-wheat bread or ⅓ cup cooked brown rice.) And it appears that greater whole-grain intake is associated with less obesity, diabetes, high blood pressure, and high cholesterol. All grains start out as whole grains, but they only remain that way if, after processing, they still contain all three whole-grain components: the germ, the endosperm, and the bran. The bran is full of fiber, while the germ and endosperm have many of the phytonutrients—beneficial chemicals found in plant foods. For example, a bran cereal may be loaded with fiber when compared to a whole-grain flaked cereal because the bran cereal contains only the wheat's fiber-loaded bran. But the bran cereal, although still a healthy choice, won't necessarily have all of the beneficial antioxidants or compounds that the whole-grain cereal offers. See page 69 to find out more about identifying whole-grain foods in the grocery store.

6. Go fish.

The American Heart Association recommends that adults eat at least 6 ounces of cooked fish per week as part of a healthful diet that can help lower the risk of heart disease. Fish, like meat, is high in protein, but it doesn't carry the high levels of saturated fat. And certain types of fatty fish like salmon and trout offer beneficial omega-3 fatty acids. This type of fat is linked with lowering triglycerides, which likely reduces blood-clot risks and prevents abnormal heart rhythms. It may also slow plaque buildup on artery walls. (See page 94 for more information about the types of fish that contain high levels of omega-3s and other fish-related health information.)

our guide to the healthiest eating, continued

7. Eat your beans and legumes.

Beans and legumes are low in fat and calories and are good sources of protein, folate, fiber, and antioxidants. In fact, these vegetables are so important, the USDA's Dietary Guidelines recommend consuming three cups of cooked beans each week. A cup of cooked black beans provides about one-third of your daily protein needs, more than 60% of the recommended amount of folate, one-fifth of your iron needs, a good dose of potassium, and 15 grams of fiber in a complex carbohydrate package. Beans and legumes may also help manage and prevent type 2 diabetes, promote cardiac health, and reduce the risk for some digestive tract cancers.

8. Use MyPyramid.

The USDA's MyPyramid provides Americans with healthy eating guidelines. Those recommendations are included at the start of each chapter, but in general, it advises Americans to eat more fruits and vegetables, consume three servings of low-fat dairy and three or more servings of whole grains daily, and maintain a moderate intake of healthful fats, such as those found in olive oil, nuts, and avocados. A staircase reminds users to stay active. The pyramid is Web-based, allowing users to tailor it to their needs based on age, gender, height, weight, and activity levels. Check it out at www.mypyramid.gov.

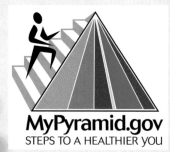

how to use this book

Throughout this guide, we've used some icons and phrases regularly to denote what's healthy and what's unhealthy. (We've also included glossaries of nutrition terms, vitamins, and minerals starting on page 324 to help you.) Here's what you'll find:

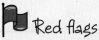 Red flags

The red flags and the use of the color red denote things to watch out for in the grocery store. The flags are also used to indicate certain phrases on a label to be aware of or something you should look out for in the ingredient list.

The color green

We used green throughout to highlight how to choose and find the good-for-you things in the grocery store.

Yellow highlights

All the information in this book is important, but we've used yellow highlights to help you spot the most important information.

The phrase "a good source of"

This term denotes those foods that provide 10% to 19% of the recommended daily amount of a particular vitamin, mineral, or nutrient.

The phrase "an excellent source of"

This term denotes those foods that provide 20% or more of the recommended daily amount of a particular vitamin, mineral, or nutrient.

fresh produce

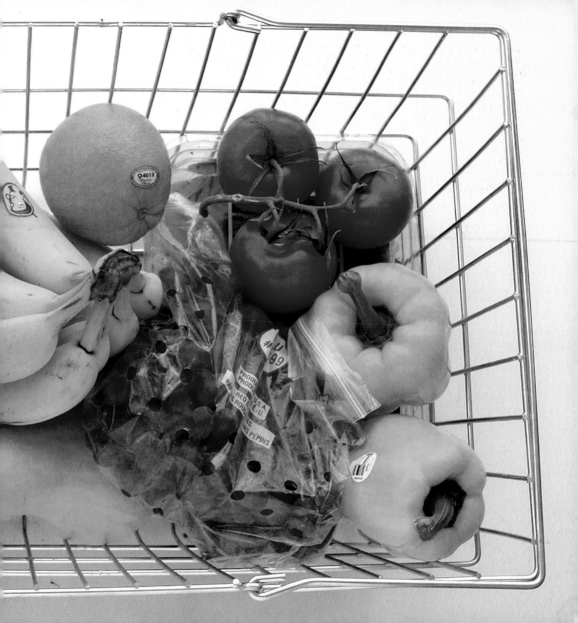

fresh produce

Why eat fruits and vegetables?

Fruits and vegetables:
- ☑ are low in calories
- ☑ are high in fiber
- ☑ are packed with vitamins, minerals, and antioxidants
- ☑ help prevent heart disease and stroke
- ☑ help control blood pressure
- ☑ ward off certain cancers
- ☑ protect vision
- ☑ help the gastrointestinal tract stay healthy

How much should I eat?

The USDA's Dietary Guidelines recommend adults eat anywhere from 5 to 13 servings of fruits and vegetables per day depending on age, gender, physical activity, and overall health.

Use your fist to approximate a fruit or vegetable serving—a fist is about 1 cup.

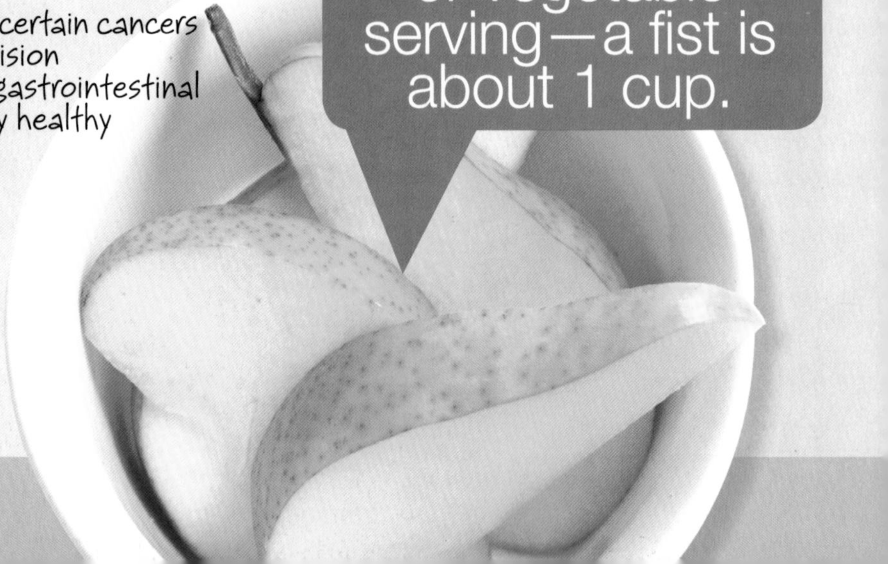

What is a serving?

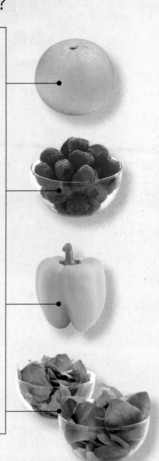

1 small apple = 1 serving

1 large orange = 1 serving

1 banana = 1 serving

1 cup berries or grapes = 1 serving

1 cup raw fruits or vegetables = 1 serving

1 small bell pepper = ½ serving

1 cup cooked squash = 1 serving

2 cups leafy greens = 1 serving

choose the
healthiest produce

Fruits and vegetables are among the most nutritious foods you can eat. In fact, none are bad for you, and all offer a host of health benefits.

1. Whole fruits and vegetables are best.

When you eat fresh fruit and vegetables in their original forms, you reap the most nutritional benefits. For produce with an edible skin, eat the skin, too. While you still get the vitamins, minerals, and antioxidants from produce in its frozen, canned, dried, and juice forms, you miss out on the important effects of fiber. Fiber not only helps keep you feeling fuller longer, but it also aids in heart and digestive health.

2. Choose colorful produce.

The vitamins and phytochemicals that give fruits and vegetables their colors work as antioxidants, immune boosters, and anti-inflammatories. The best way to obtain them is to eat a variety of fresh produce based on color. The deeper the color, the more phytonutrients they contain.

3. White fruits and vegetables are also good for you.

Produce in every hue offers nutritional benefits, even white ones such as cauliflower, onions, and garlic. Like their colorful cousins, these paler versions also contain good-for-you compounds that have been linked to cancer prevention.

Watch out for added sugar in fruit that is not raw.

While all forms of fruits and vegetables are good for you, watch out for extra calories and sugar in frozen, canned, dried, and juice forms. Dried fruits and fruit juices often contain more calories than fresh whole fruits and vegetables and may have less, if any, fiber.

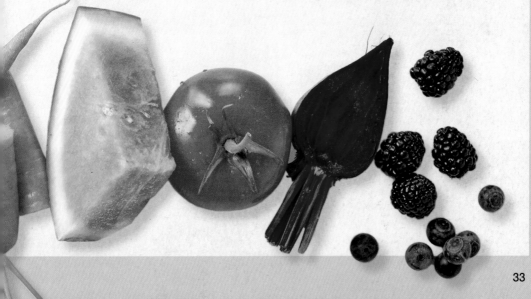

33

choose the healthiest organic produce

If you want to buy organic produce but don't want to pay the premium price for everything on your shopping list, follow these guidelines.

skip organic for these fruits and vegetables

These are the top five fruits and the top five vegetables least likely to contain trace levels of pesticides, so feel free to buy conventional.

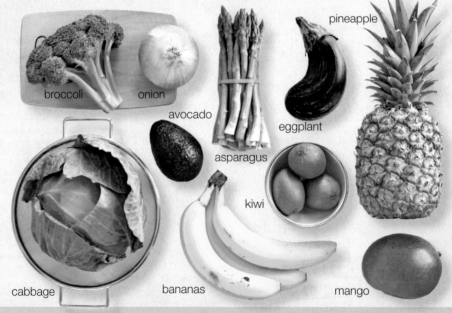

broccoli

onion

avocado

asparagus

pineapple

eggplant

kiwi

cabbage

bananas

mango

best produce to buy organic

The fruits and vegetables below are among those most likely to contain trace levels of pesticides, so consider buying organic when possible.

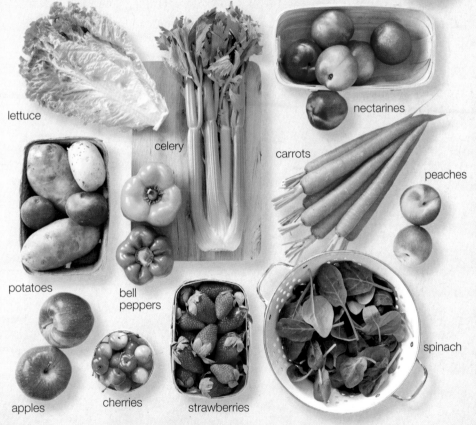

lettuce

celery

nectarines

carrots

peaches

potatoes

bell peppers

apples

cherries

strawberries

spinach

This is the recommended amount of fruits and vegetables most people should eat daily.

fruits

apples

benefits
- fiber
- vitamin C
- antioxidants

fyi
Put down your peeler. A medium Red Delicious apple with the skin on has about twice as much fiber and 45% more antioxidants than a peeled apple.

apricots

benefits
- vitamin A
- vitamin C
- fiber
- potassium

fyi
Apricots are one of the best sources of beta-carotene, which is converted to vitamin A in the body. One fresh apricot provides about the daily recommendation.

avocado

benefits
- heart-healthy unsaturated fats
- folate
- potassium
- vitamin E

bananas

benefits
- potassium
- fiber
- vitamin C
- vitamin B_6

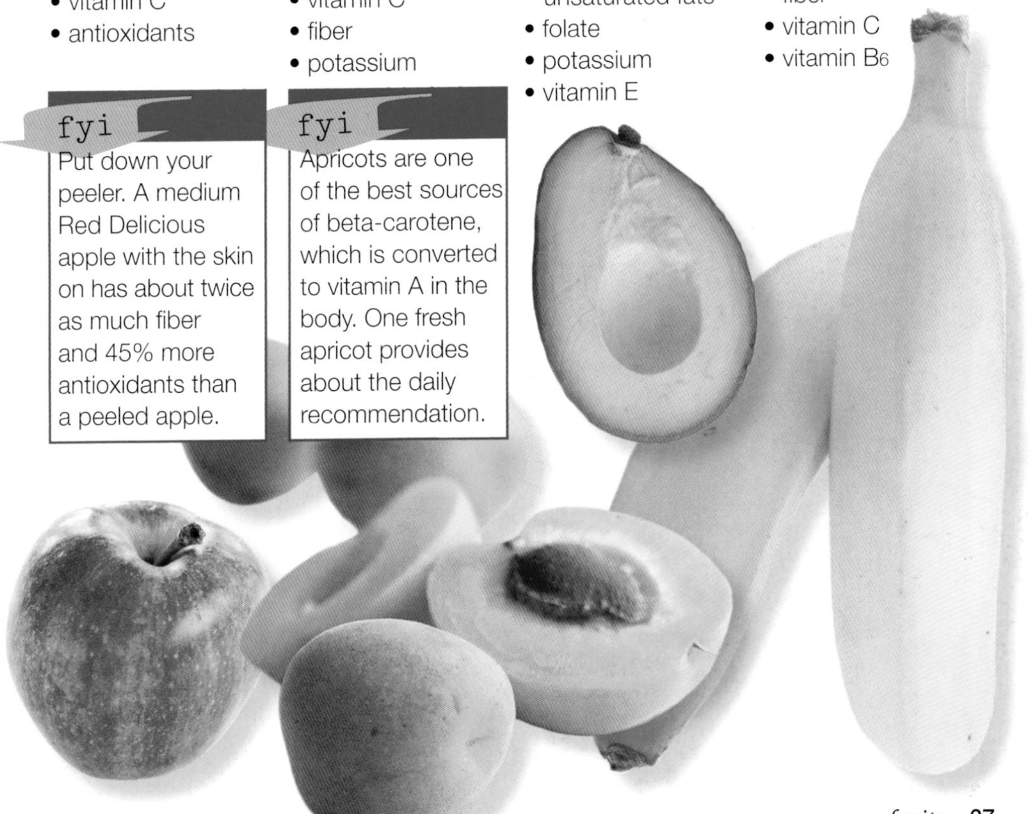

fruits, berries
continued

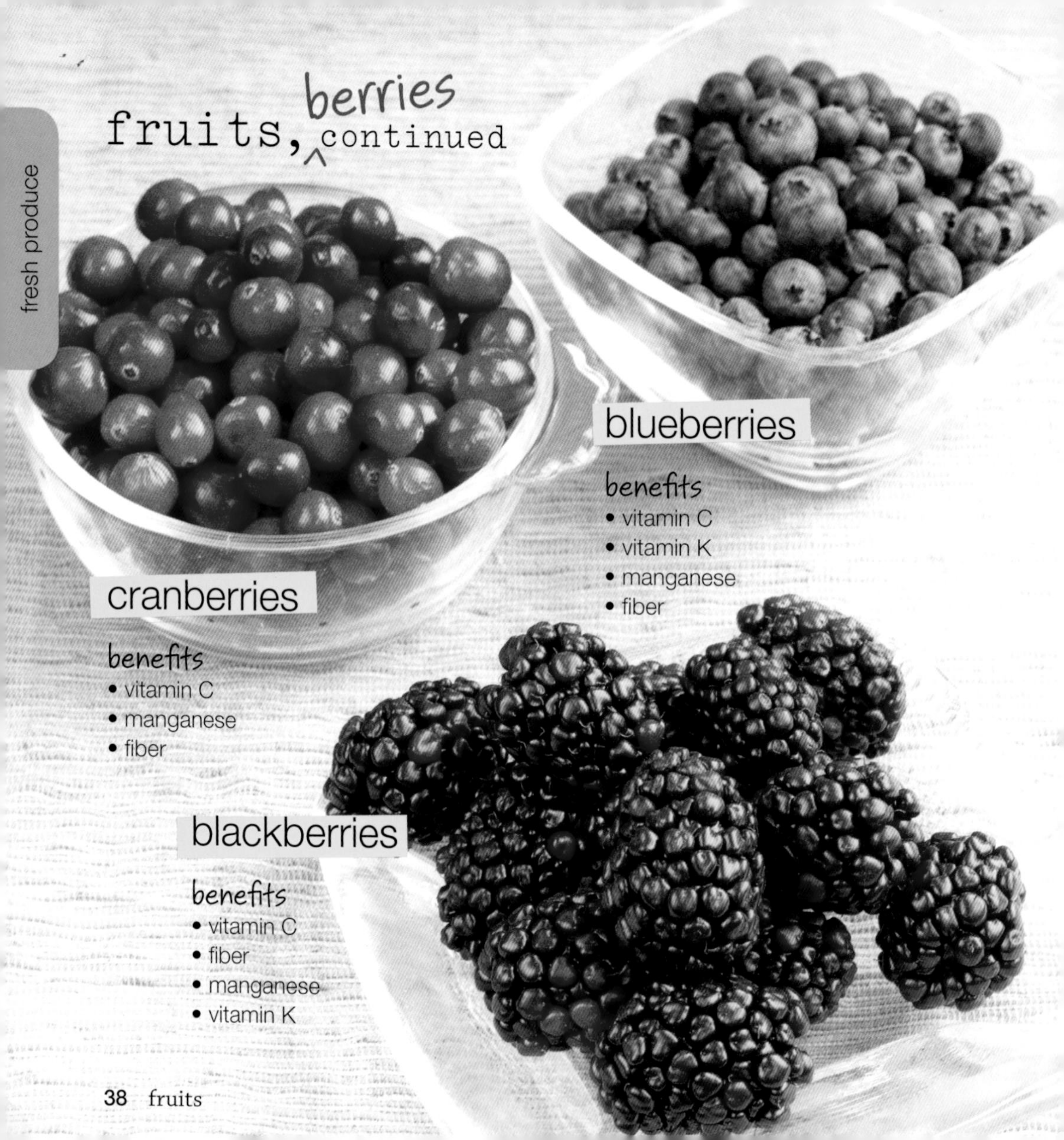

blueberries

benefits
- vitamin C
- vitamin K
- manganese
- fiber

cranberries

benefits
- vitamin C
- manganese
- fiber

blackberries

benefits
- vitamin C
- fiber
- manganese
- vitamin K

raspberries

benefits
- fiber
- vitamin C
- manganese
- vitamin K

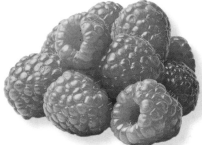

What's so great about berries?

Berries are as healthful as they are delicious. They are packed with antioxidants that offer a host of health benefits. They are also storehouses of fiber; vitamins A, C, and E; folic acid; and the minerals potassium and calcium. And they contain ellagic acid and lignans, plant compounds that may reduce the risk of some cancers.

cherries

benefits
- vitamin C
- fiber
- potassium

strawberries

benefits
- vitamin C
- manganese
- fiber

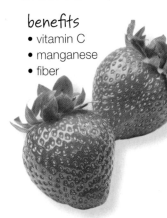

fruits, *citrus* continued

lemons and limes

benefits
• vitamin C

Citrus fruits have vitamin C, which may reduce the risk of cancer and cataracts.

grapefruit

benefits
- fiber
- vitamin C

fyi
The pink and red varieties of grapefruit are an excellent source of vitamin A and lycopene.

oranges

benefits
- vitamin C
- fiber
- folate

fyi
The more of the white part of an orange you eat, the more fiber you get.

tangerines

benefits
- vitamin C
- fiber

fyi
Among citrus fruits, the tangerine is the highest in pectin, a fiber that makes you feel fuller.

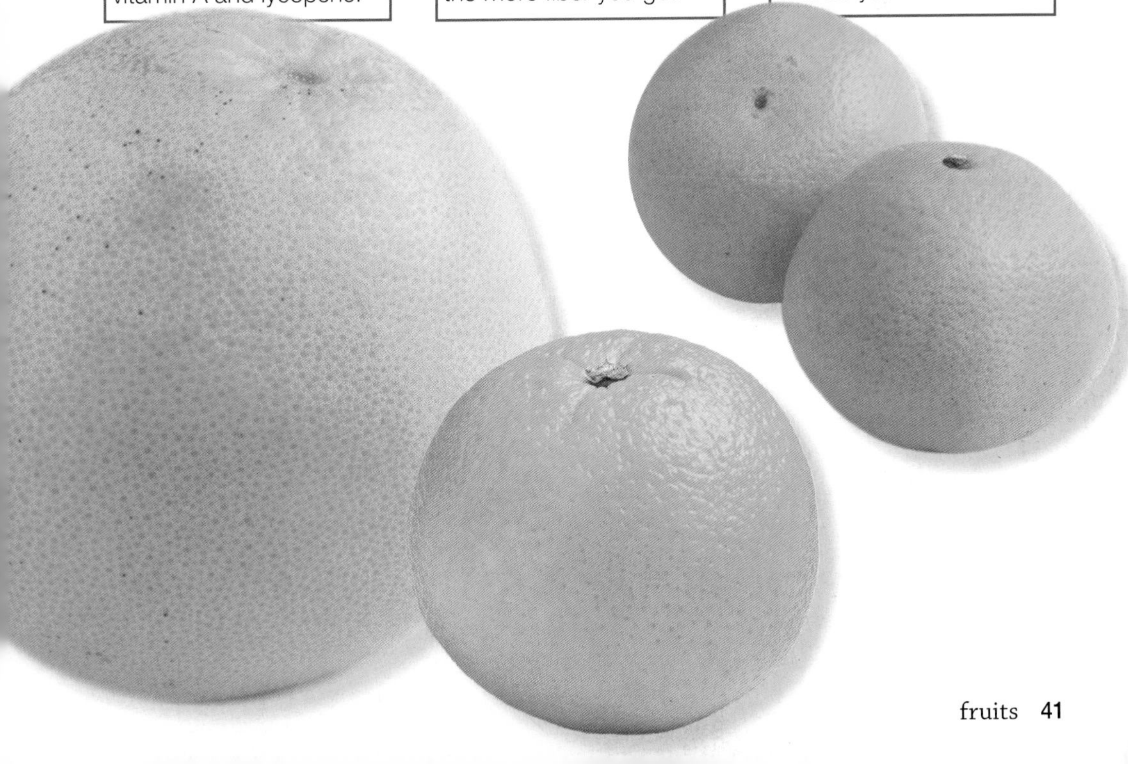

fruits, continued

figs

benefits
- fiber
- iron
- calcium
- potassium

grapes

benefits
- vitamin C
- manganese
- vitamin K

kiwi

benefits
- vitamin C
- vitamin K
- fiber
- potassium

mangoes

benefits
- vitamin C
- vitamin A
- beta-carotene

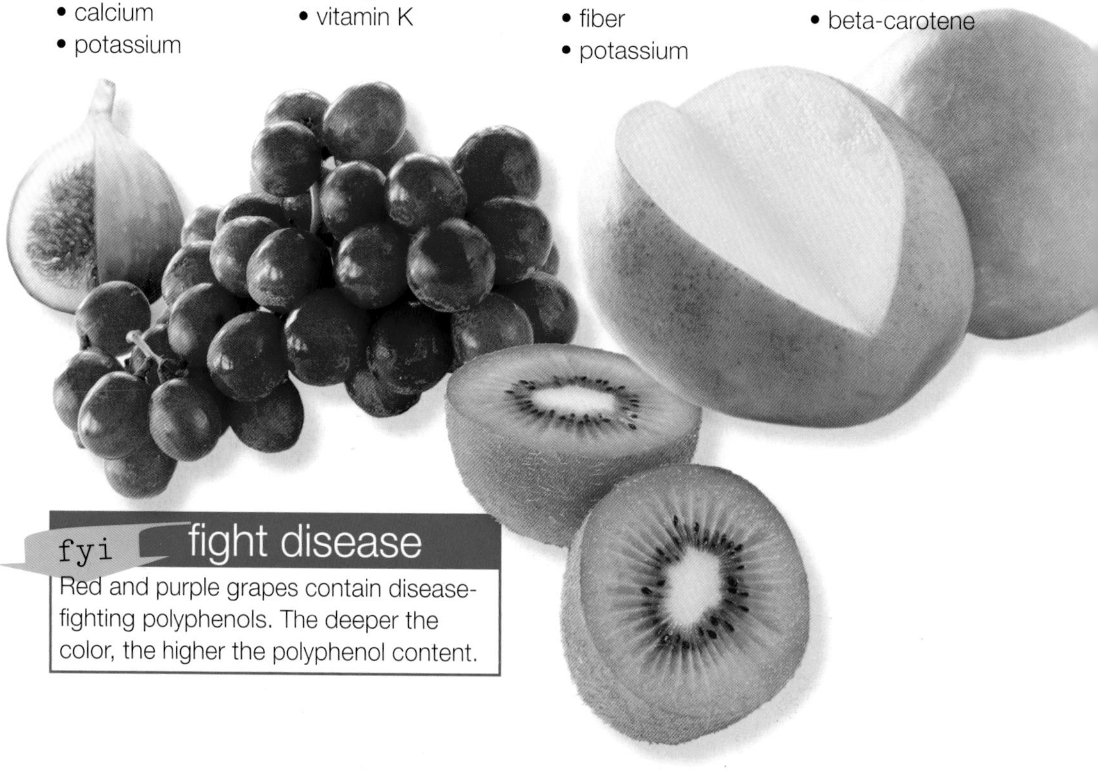

fyi fight disease
Red and purple grapes contain disease-fighting polyphenols. The deeper the color, the higher the polyphenol content.

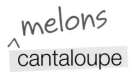

melons

cantaloupe

benefits
- vitamin A
- vitamin C
- potassium

honeydew

benefits
- vitamin C
- potassium

watermelon

benefits
- vitamin A
- vitamin C
- lycopene

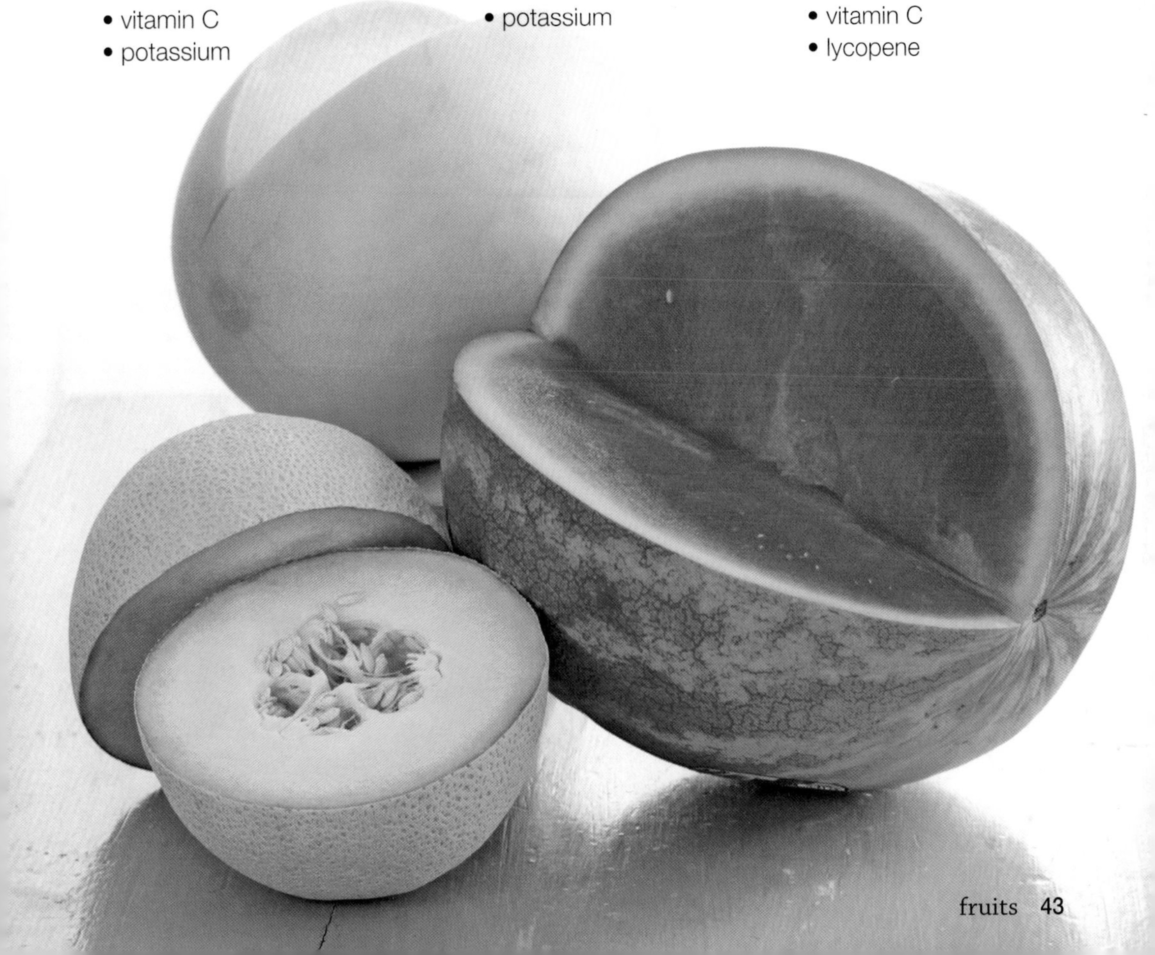

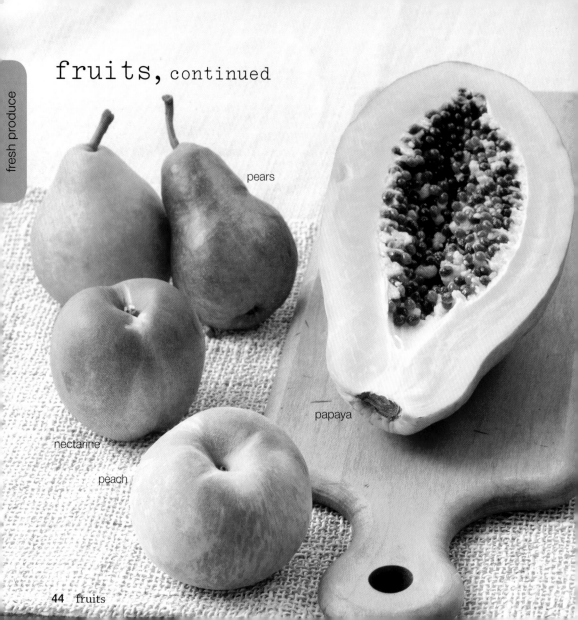

fruits, continued

pears

papaya

nectarine

peach

nectarines

benefits
- vitamin C

peaches

benefits
- vitamin C

believe it or not...

Nectarines and peaches are so closely related that, though rare, you can sometimes find them growing on the same tree.

pears

benefits
- fiber
- vitamin C

fyi

One medium pear contains 4 grams of fiber—most of it is in the peel.

papaya

benefits
- vitamin C
- vitamin A
- fiber
- folate
- potassium

pineapple

benefits
- vitamin C
- manganese

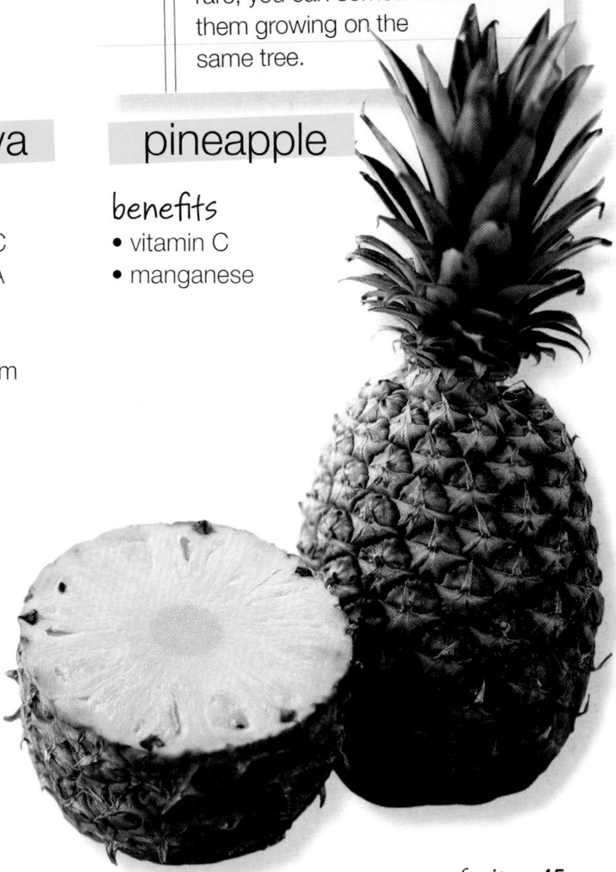

fruits, continued

plums

benefits
- vitamin C
- vitamin K

dried plums (prunes)

benefits
- fiber
- iron
- vitamin K

pomegranate

benefits
- potassium
- vitamin C

raisins

benefits
- potassium
- fiber

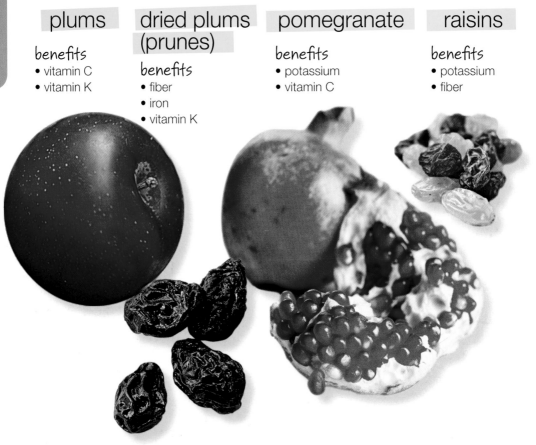

vegetables

artichokes

benefits
- fiber
- vitamin C
- vitamin K
- folate
- magnesium
- potassium
- manganese

asparagus

benefits
- folate
- vitamin K
- vitamin C
- vitamin A

fyi

White asparagus lacks heart-protecting phytonutrients and provides less of vitamins A and C compared to its green counterpart.

beets

benefits
- folate
- manganese
- fiber
- potassium

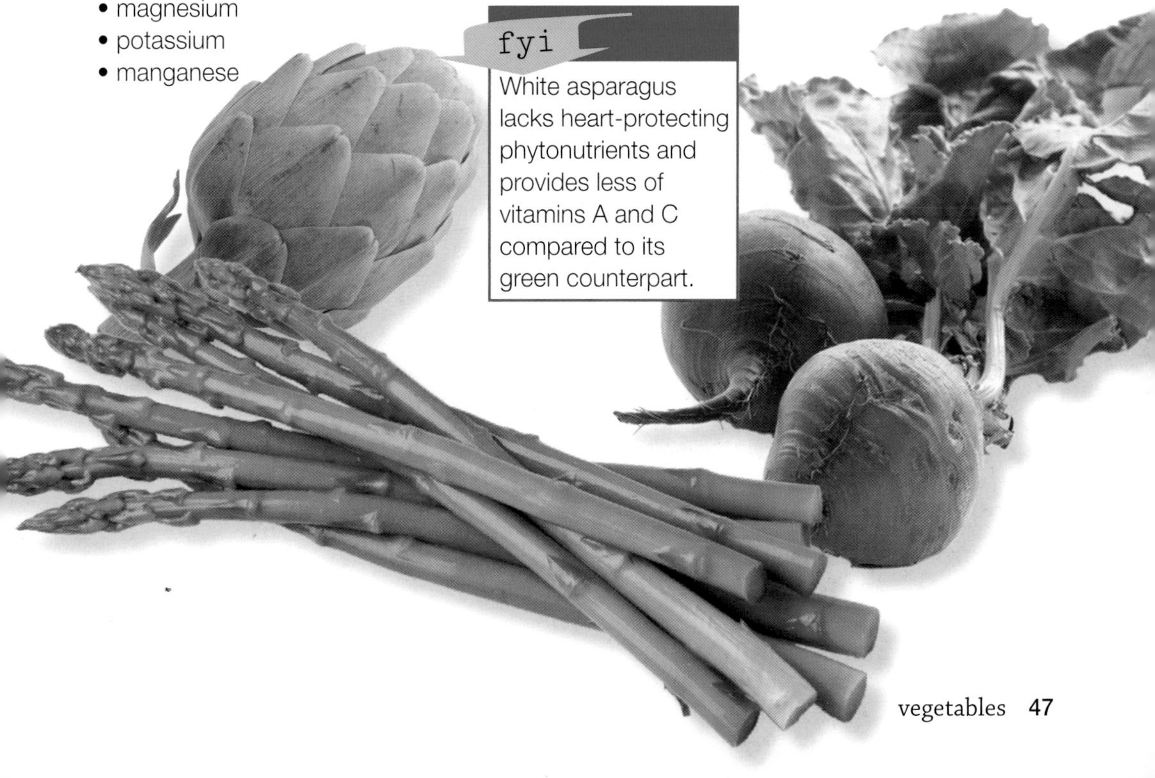

vegetables, beans continued

beans

benefits
- rich in protein
- fiber
- folate
- potassium
- iron

edamame (green soybeans)

benefits
- heart-healthy fats
- rich in protein
- fiber
- folate
- potassium
- iron

green beans

benefits
- fiber
- vitamin K
- vitamin A
- vitamin C
- potassium
- folate

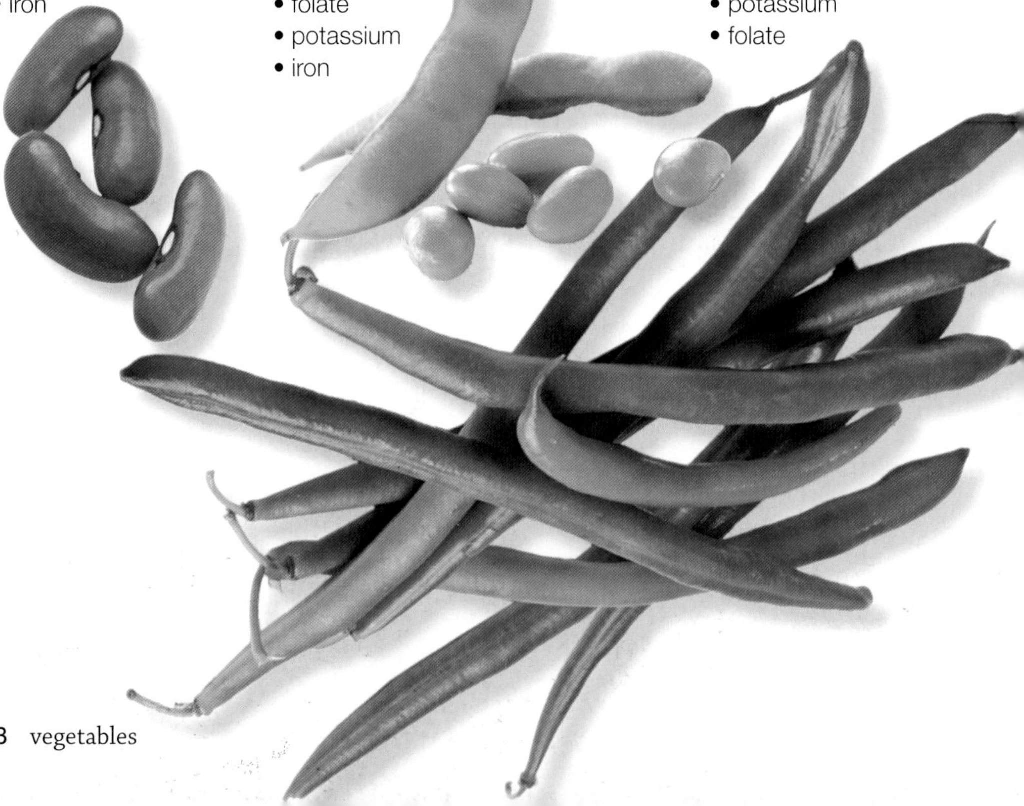

bell peppers

benefits
- vitamin C
- vitamin E
- vitamin A
- vitamin B6
- fiber

vegetables, continued

Brussels sprouts

benefits
- folate
- vitamin A
- vitamin C
- vitamin K
- fiber
- iron
- potassium
- beta-carotene

cabbage

benefits
- vitamin K
- vitamin C

fyi
Red cabbage is a good source of folate, while green is a good source of vitamin B6 and manganese.

carrots

benefits
- vitamin A
- vitamin K
- potassium
- lutein
- beta-carotene

broccoli

benefits
- vitamin C
- vitamin K
- folate
- fiber
- vitamin A
- vitamin B6
- potassium
- riboflavin
- manganese

cauliflower

benefits
- vitamin C
- vitamin K
- folate
- vitamin B6
- fiber
- contains cancer-fighting indoles and isothiocyanates

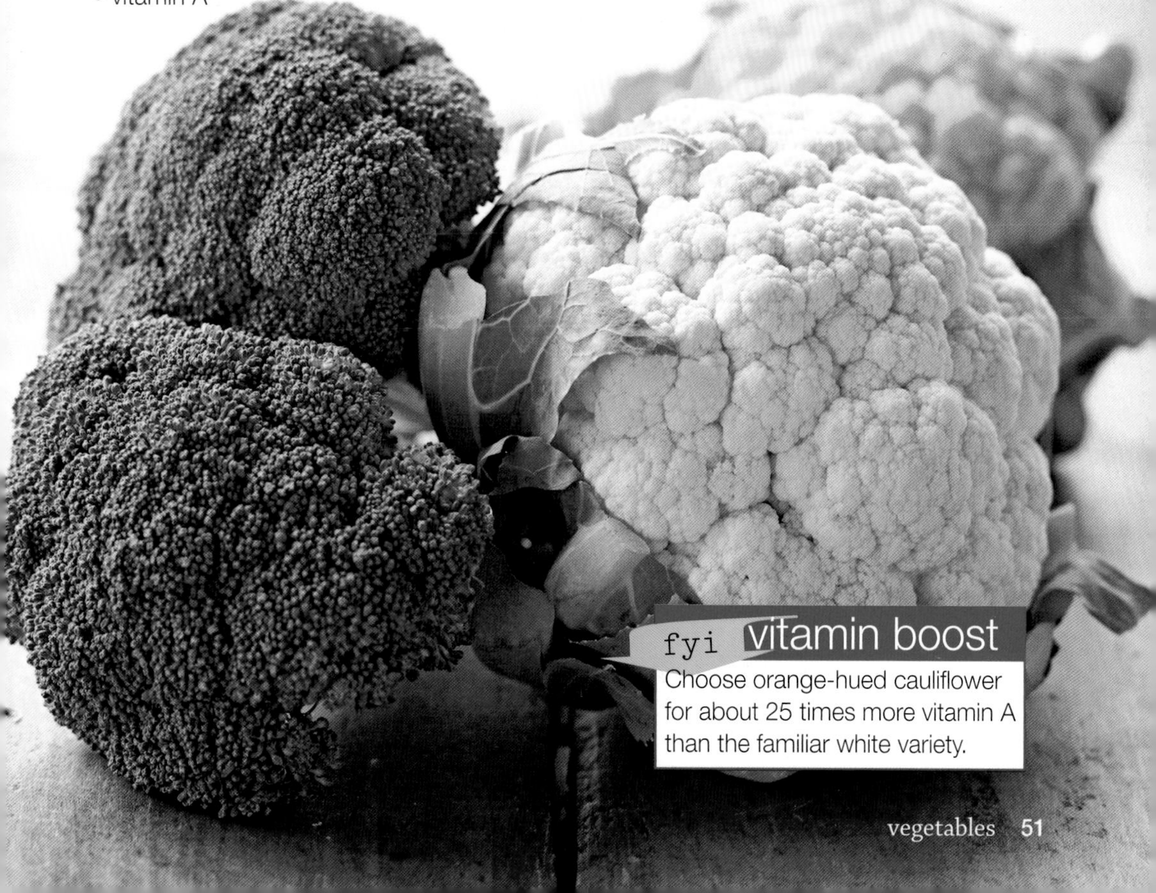

fyi vitamin boost
Choose orange-hued cauliflower for about 25 times more vitamin A than the familiar white variety.

vegetables, continued

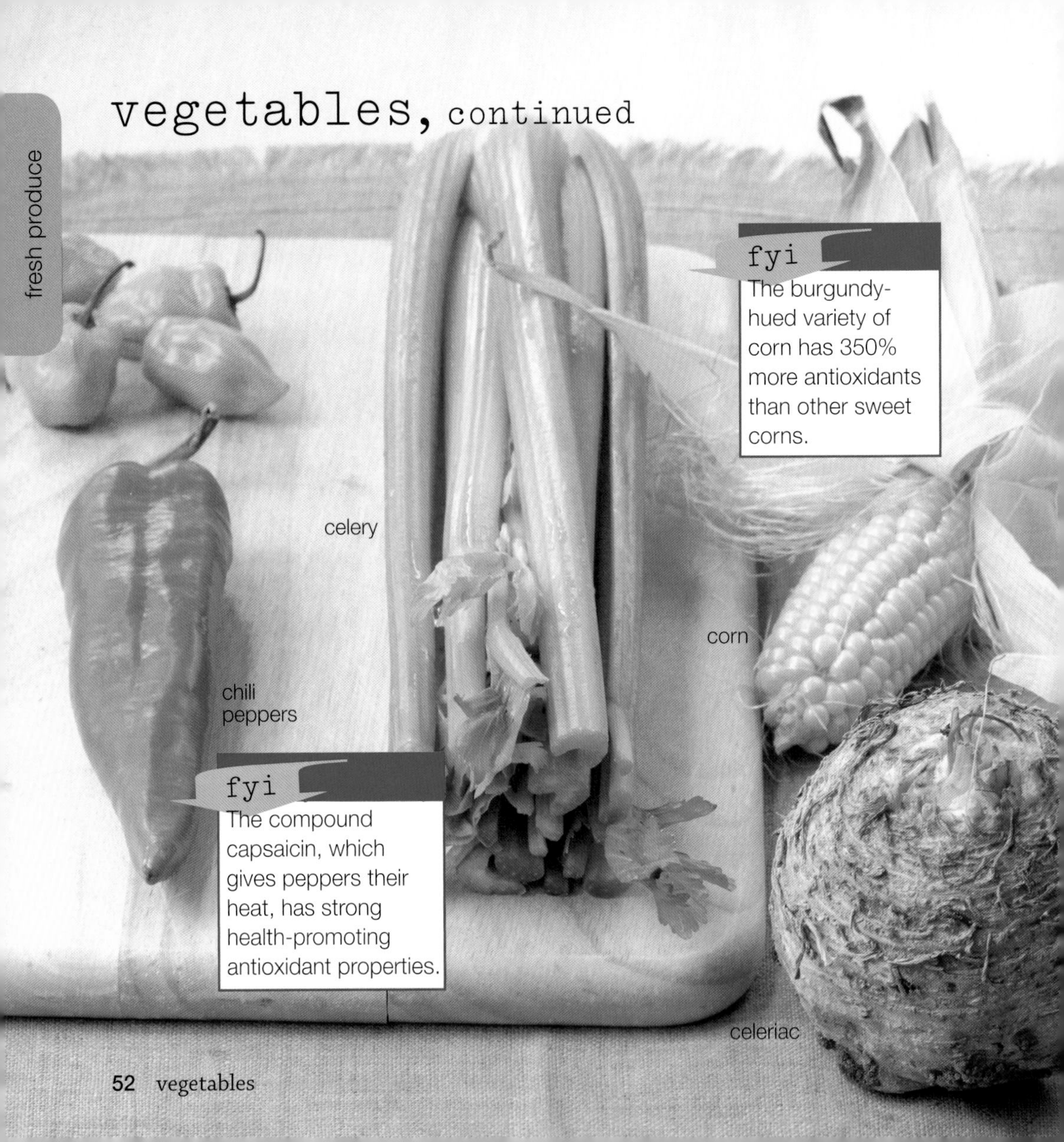

fyi
The burgundy-hued variety of corn has 350% more antioxidants than other sweet corns.

celery

corn

chili peppers

fyi
The compound capsaicin, which gives peppers their heat, has strong health-promoting antioxidant properties.

celeriac

celeriac

benefits
- fiber
- potassium

celery

benefits
- vitamin K
- vitamin C
- folate
- potassium

chili peppers

benefits
- vitamin C

corn

benefits
- fiber
- folate
- potassium
- vitamin C

cucumbers

benefits
- vitamin K

eggplant

benefits
- fiber

fennel

benefits
- vitamin C

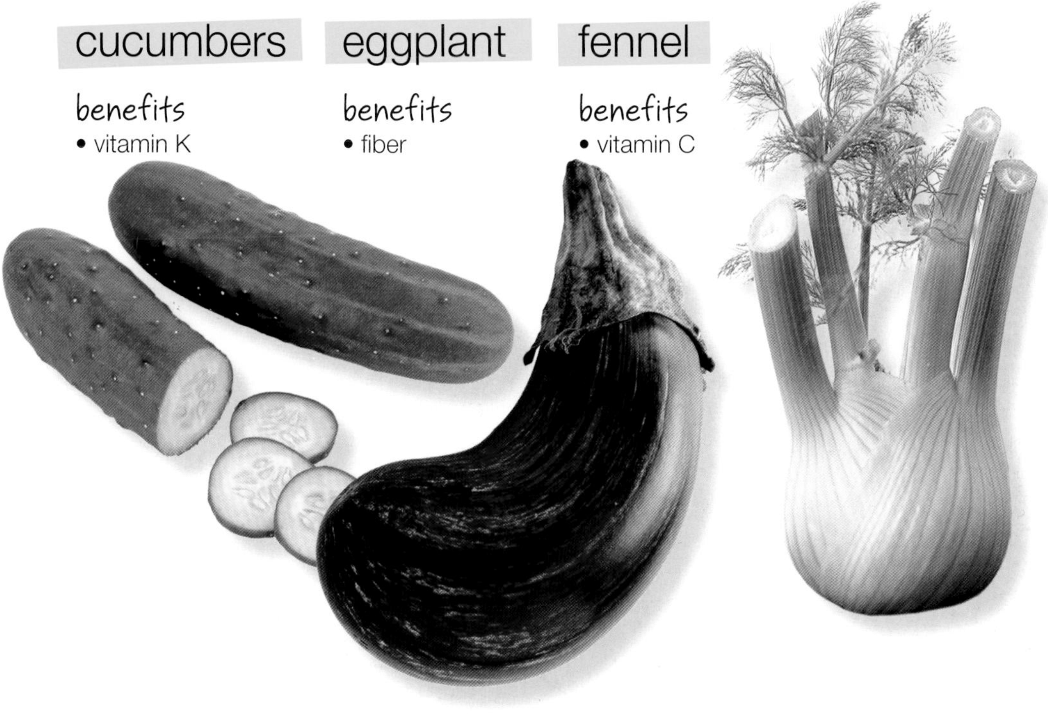

vegetables, ^{greens} continued

leafy greens

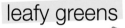

benefits
- vitamin A
- vitamin K
- fiber
- folate
- antioxidants, including beta-carotene and lutein

arugula

radicchio

frisée

endive

escarole

iceberg

romaine

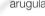
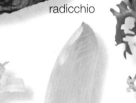

The greener the lettuce, the more nutrients, vitamins, and minerals it contains.

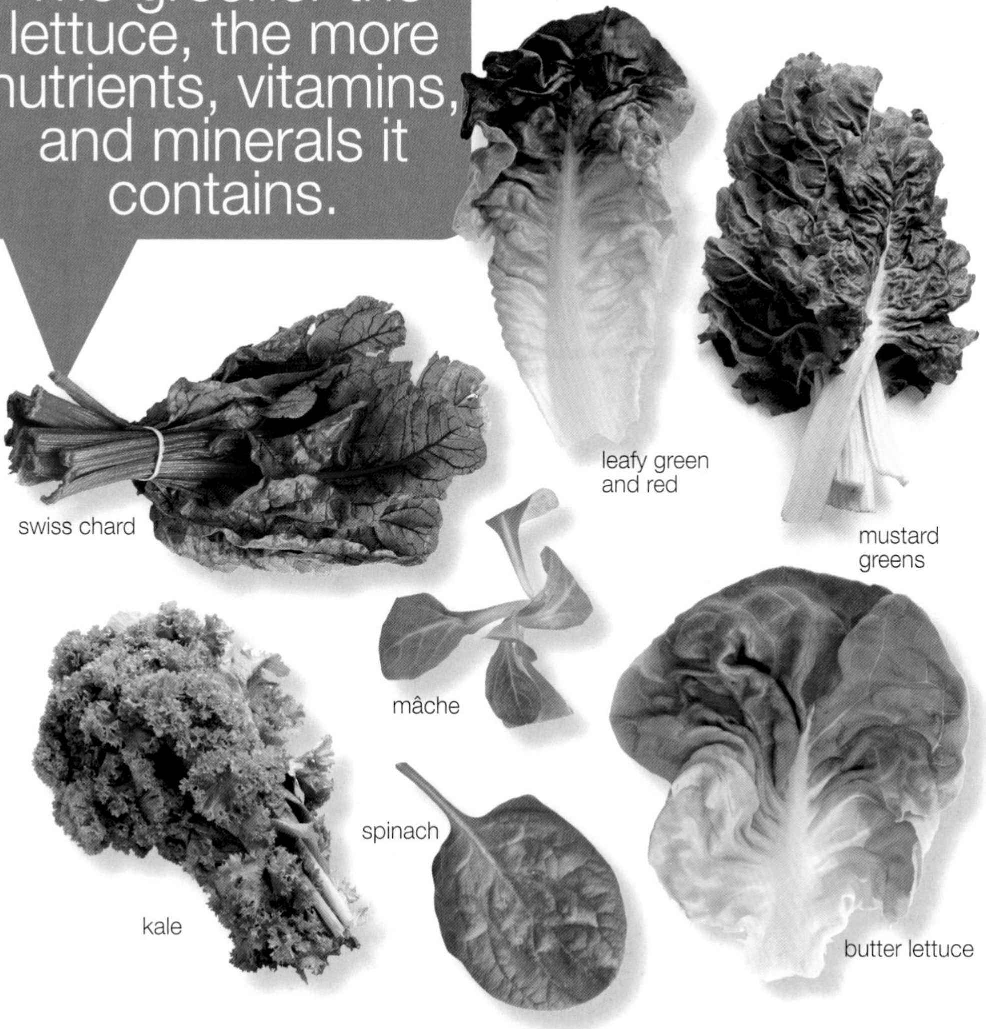

swiss chard

leafy green and red

mustard greens

mâche

kale

spinach

butter lettuce

vegetables, continued

jicama

benefits
- fiber
- vitamin C

leeks

benefits
- vitamin A
- manganese

mushrooms

benefits
- riboflavin
- niacin
- potassium
- antioxidants

okra

benefits
- vitamin C
- folate
- fiber

onions

benefits
- vitamin C
- vitamin B6
- fiber
- manganese

Q&A Do mushrooms have any nutritional value?

Mushrooms are 90% water and have only 18 calories per cup, but they harbor large amounts of antioxidants. They also offer a healthy dose of potassium, which plays a role in lowering blood pressure.

vegetables, continued

peas

benefits
- vitamin C
- vitamin A
- folate
- fiber
- protein

potatoes

benefits

- potassium
- vitamin C
- fiber
- magnesium
- manganese
- niacin
- vitamin B6
- folate

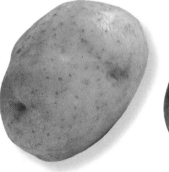

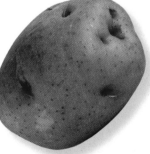

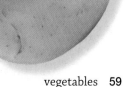

vegetables, continued

parsnips

benefits
- fiber
- potassium
- vitamin C
- folate

radishes

benefits
- vitamin C

rhubarb

benefits
- vitamin K
- fiber
- potassium
- vitamin C
- manganese

^squash

acorn squash

benefits
- fiber
- potassium
- vitamin B6
- magnesium

butternut squash

benefits
- vitamin A
- vitamin C
- vitamin E
- fiber
- potassium

pumpkin

benefits
- vitamin A
- vitamin C
- potassium
- fiber
- lutein

zucchini

benefits
- vitamin C
- vitamin B6
- potassium
- fiber
- lutein

yellow summer squash

benefits
- vitamin C
- vitamin B6
- potassium
- fiber
- lutein

vegetables, continued

sweet potatoes

benefits

- vitamin A
- fiber
- vitamin C
- potassium
- manganese
- beta-carotene

tomatoes

benefits

- vitamin A
- vitamin C
- vitamin K
- potassium
- lycopene

turnips

benefits

- fiber
- vitamin C

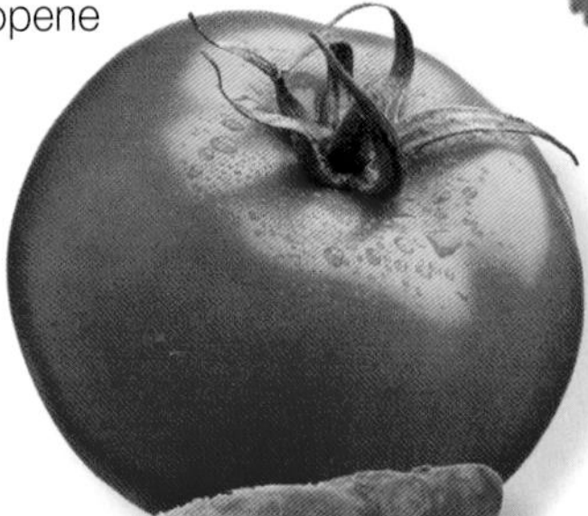

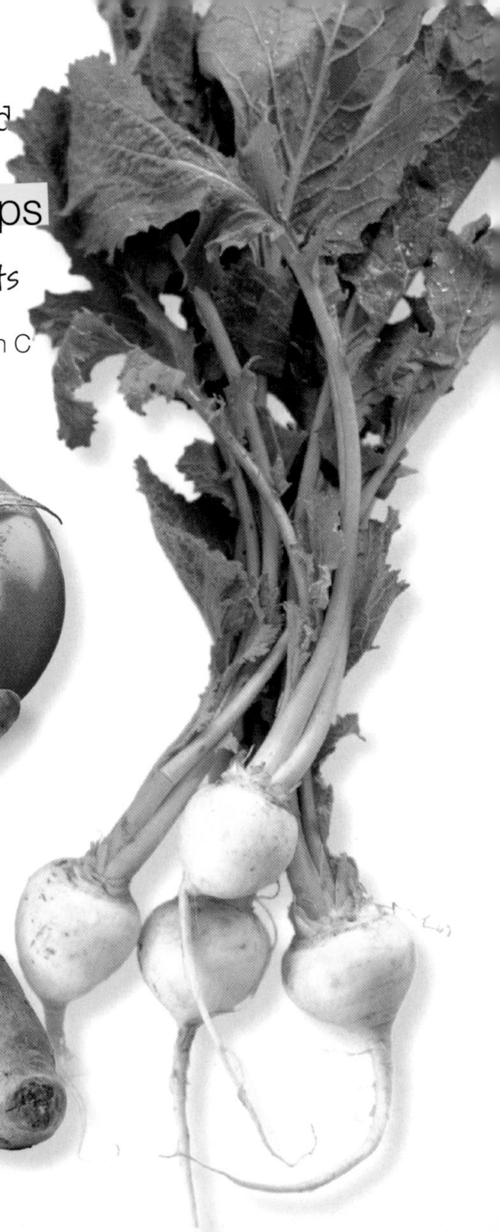

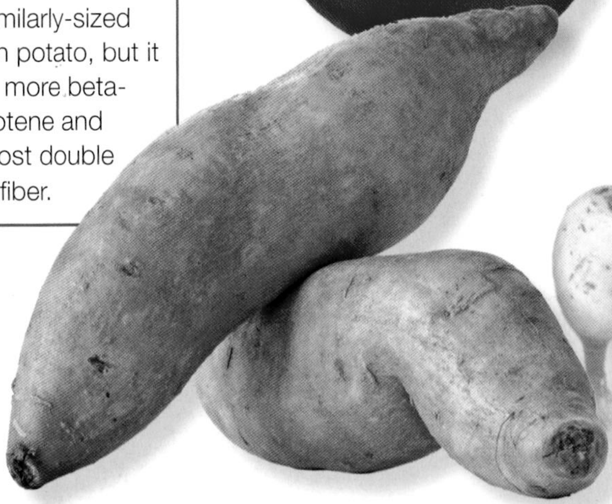

fyi

A sweet potato contains slightly more calories than a similarly-sized plain potato, but it has more beta-carotene and almost double the fiber.

herbs

fresh herbs

benefits
- vitamin A
- vitamin C
- vitamin K

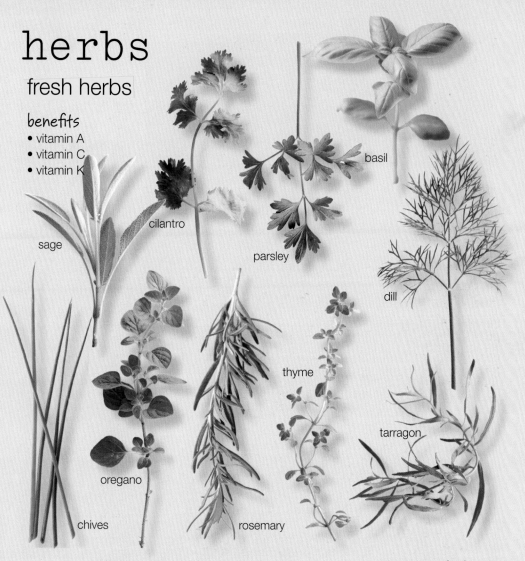

sage

cilantro

parsley

basil

dill

oregano

thyme

tarragon

chives

rosemary

breads

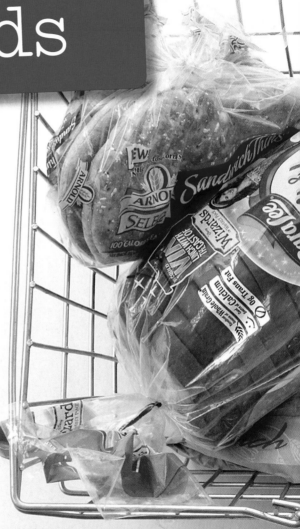

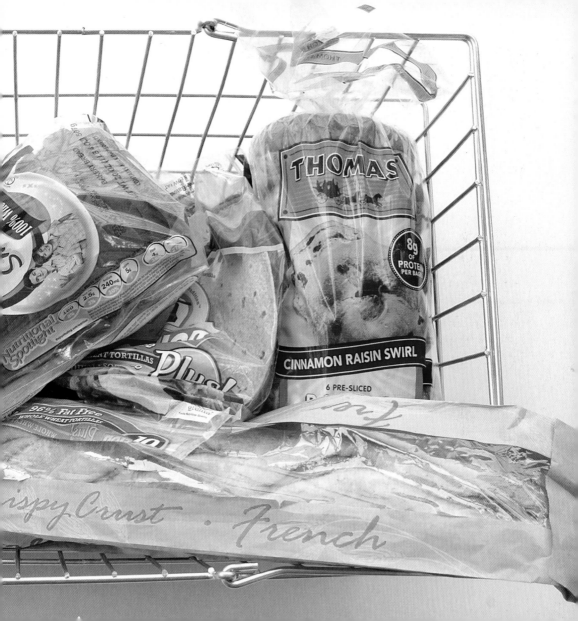

breads

Why eat breads?
The healthiest breads contain:
- ☑ whole grains
- ☑ fiber
- ☑ protein
- ☑ vitamin B6
- ☑ vitamin E
- ☑ folic acid
- ☑ magnesium
- ☑ zinc

How much should I eat?
According to the USDA, the amount of grains you need to eat depends on your age, gender, and level of physical activity. Most adults and children need 5 to 8 servings per day.

At least half of all the grains eaten on a daily basis should be whole grains.

What is a serving?

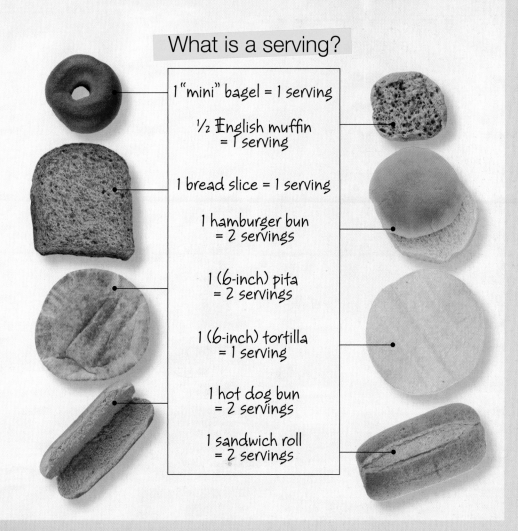

1 "mini" bagel = 1 serving

½ English muffin = 1 serving

1 bread slice = 1 serving

1 hamburger bun = 2 servings

1 (6-inch) pita = 2 servings

1 (6-inch) tortilla = 1 serving

1 hot dog bun = 2 servings

1 sandwich roll = 2 servings

choose the ==healthiest== breads

All breads are not created equal, but there are some common elements that all healthy breads share. Here's what to look for no matter what type of bread you're shopping for.

1. When deciding between two similar bread products, look at the calories and fiber.

A low fiber content is a sign that processing has stripped the bread of this nutrient, which means other valuable nutrients could also be missing. Follow the guidelines we've outlined throughout the chapter for specific bread products.

2. Look for breads that don't contain a lot of sugar.

Too much sugar means unnecessary calories have been added. The sweetener should be one of the last ingredients listed, and the grams of sugar per serving should be equal to or less than the grams of fiber.

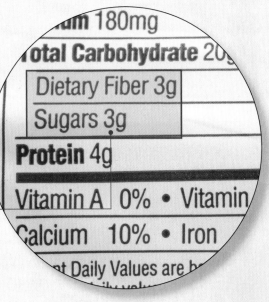

...um 180mg

Total Carbohydrate 20g

Dietary Fiber 3g

Sugars 3g

Protein 4g

Vitamin A | 0% • Vitamin

Calcium | 10% • Iron

...t Daily Values are b...

3. Choose whole grains.

Terms like "health nut," "9-grain," and "multigrain" all sound healthy, but they don't necessarily mean the breads are made with whole grains. Instead, look for "100% whole grain" or "100% whole wheat" on the package. If one of those isn't there, check the ingredient list. The first ingredient should be "whole-wheat flour," "whole grain," "whole oats," or "whole rye" instead of "enriched."

Here are two other ways to tell if the bread is whole grain:

• Look for the Food and Drug Administration–approved claim. It links consumption of whole grains to a reduced risk of heart disease and some types of cancer.

• Look for the black-and-yellow Whole Grain Stamp. The stamp, developed by the Whole Grains Council, guarantees you get at least half a serving (8 grams) of whole grains in each serving—the exact amount will be listed. The stamp can be placed anywhere on the package. This is a voluntary program, so not all whole-grain products carry it.

made with whole grain oats

Stone Ground Wheat

Diets rich in whole grain foods and other plant foods and low in total fat, saturated fat, and cholesterol, may help reduce the risk of Heart Disease and Certain Cancers.

WHOLE GRAIN RYE CRISPBREAD
All Natural Ingredients

100% WHOLE WHEAT

Baked with 100% Whole Grain

WholeGrainsCouncil.org
WHOLE GRAIN
Good Source

watch out for these red flags

There are good things to look for on a label as well as items to beware of. Here are the red flags to watch out for.

⚑ Watch out for the phrase "made with whole grains."

When a package reads "made with whole grains," it means the bread is made with a blend of whole-wheat flour and some other kind—most likely a less nutritious flour. While the bread still contains good-for-you whole grains that make it a better choice than white bread, you're not getting the most nutritional bang for your buck.

Soft MADE WITH Whole Grain White

Nutrition Facts

Serving Size 2 Slices (57g)
Servings Per Container 10

Calories 160
Calories from Fat 20

Calories Per Slice 80
Calories from Fat 10

Amount/Serving	% Daily Value* 2 SLICES 1 SLICE	
Total Fat 2g, 1g	3%	2%
Saturated Fat 0.5g, 0g	3%	0%
Trans Fat 0g, 0g		
Polyunsaturated Fat 1g, 0.5g		
Monounsaturated Fat 0g, 0g		
Cholesterol 0mg, 0mg	0%	0%
Vitamin A	0%	0%
Vitamin C	0%	0%
Calcium	10%	4%
Iron	10%	6%

Amount/Serving	% Daily Value* 2 SLICES 1 SLICE	
Sodium 270mg, 130mg	11%	5%
Total Carbohydrate 30g, 15g	10%	5%
Dietary Fiber 1g, Less than 1g	5%	2%
Sugars 4g, 2g		
Protein 5g, 2g		
Thiamin	15%	8%
Riboflavin	10%	6%
Niacin	10%	6%
Folic Acid	15%	8%

*Percent Daily Values are based on a 2,000 calorie diet. Your daily values may be higher or lower depending on your calorie needs:

		Calories:	2,000	2,500
Total Fat	Less than		65g	80g
Sat Fat	Less than		20g	25g
Cholesterol	Less than		300mg	300mg
Sodium	Less than		2,400mg	2,400mg
Total Carbohydrate			300g	375g
Dietary Fiber			25g	30g

Calories per gram:
Fat 9 • Carbohydrate 4 • Protein 4

INGREDIENTS: ENRICHED BLEACHED FLOUR (WHEAT FLOUR, MALTED BARLEY FLOUR, NIACIN, IRON, THIAMIN MONONITRATE (VITAMIN B1), RIBOFLAVIN (VITAMIN B2), FOLIC ACID), WHEY, WATER, HIGH FRUCTOSE CORN SYRUP, YEAST, DEXTROSE. CONTAINS 2% OR LESS OF EACH OF THE FOLLOWING: VEGETABLE OIL (SOYBEAN AND/OR COTTONSEED OILS), WHEAT GLUTEN, SALT, DOUGH CONDITIONERS (MAY CONTAIN ONE OR MORE OF THE FOLLOWING: MONO- AND DIGLYCERIDES, ETHOXYLATED MONO- AND DIGLYCERIDES, SODIUM STEAROYL LACTYLATE, CALCIUM PEROXIDE, DATEM, ASCORBIC ACID, AZODICARBONAMIDE, ENZYMES), GUAR GUM, DISTILLED VINEGAR, CALCIUM SULFATE, CALCIUM PROPIONATE (PRESERVATIVE), YEAST NUTRIENTS (MONOCALCIUM PHOSPHATE, CALCIUM SULFATE, AMMONIUM SULFATE AND/OR CALCIUM CARBONATE), CORN STARCH, SOY LECITHIN, SOY FLOUR.
CONTAINS WHEAT, MILK AND SOY
SARA LEE. DOWNERS GROVE, IL 60515 USA   © 2009 SARA LEE CORPORATION

11611-0619-1208

⚑ Watch out for enriched flour.

Enriched flour means the grain has been processed, which removes the fiber, essential fatty acids, and most of the vitamins and minerals. When breads are enriched, it's an attempt to add back some of those nutrients. While dozens of nutrients may have been removed during processing, only five, by law, have to be added back. The fiber content is lost in processing and can't be added back.

⚑ Watch out for bleached flour.

Avoid products that include bleached flour in the ingredient list. Bleaching adds chemicals to the breads while also destroying the pigments in the flour. Those pigments are beta-carotene, which your body converts into vitamin A.

ENRICHED BLEACHED FLOUR [
ONTAINS 2% OR LESS OF EACH
ETHOXYLATED MONO- AND D
SERVATIVE), YEAST NUT
ILK AND SOY

bagels

Bagels come in a wide variety of flavors, but which ones are best? Here's what you need to know.

calories

- Large bagels should have 250 calories or less per bagel.
- "Mini" bagels should have 75 calories or less per bagel.

fiber

- Large bagels should have 5 grams or more per bagel.
- "Mini" bagels should have 2 grams or more per bagel.

Watch your toppings. Bagels with full-fat cream cheese can hold as much saturated fat as a doughnut.

1 "mini" bagel = 1 serving ————————

1 large bagel = 4 servings ————

Q&A What is a proper bagel serving size?

If you're following the USDA serving-size guidelines, one serving is one "mini" bagel. The common portion you'll find in the bakery and on the supermarket aisle is much larger and can be equal to four or five servings. It's fine to have larger bagels—just know that they count more towards the daily recommendation of 5 to 8 servings. Also, look to the calorie and fiber levels (page 72) to guide you.

breads

fyi — bakery bagels

The bakery usually has lots of healthy bagel choices, but these bagels often don't come with nutrition information. If they do, follow the calorie and fiber guidelines on page 72. If not, look for these two things:

1. Check the ingredient list. The first ingredient should be whole grain (see page 69). You can also look for other good-for-you ingredients like seeds, flax, and wheat germ. These added healthy ingredients mean more calories, but the benefits—vitamins, minerals, fiber, healthy fats—can outweigh the extra calories. If you're buying from a specialty bagel shop that doesn't list the ingredients, ask the baker.

2. Watch the portion size. Bakery bagels can sometimes be supersized.

Q&A How healthy are flavored bagels?

You may be able to find some flavored bagels—cinnamon raisin, blueberry, poppy seed—that fit the nutritional bill. Just watch the sugar content so that one bagel doesn't become dessert, and be sure to follow the calorie and fiber guidelines outlined on page 72.

How healthy is your bagel?

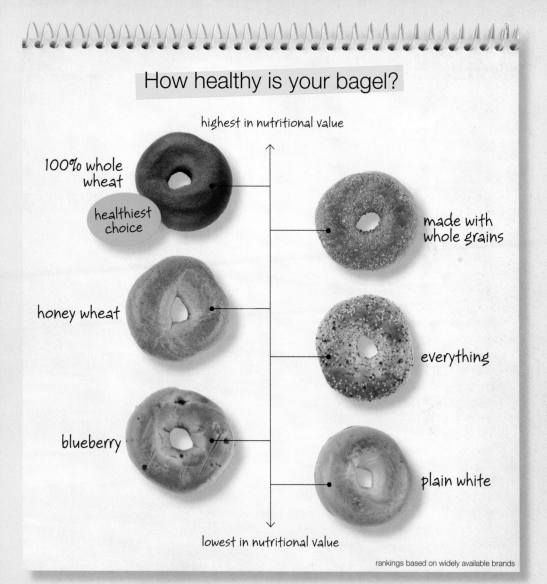

highest in nutritional value

100% whole wheat

healthiest choice

made with whole grains

honey wheat

everything

blueberry

plain white

lowest in nutritional value

rankings based on widely available brands

buns

Hamburgers and hot dogs are perennial favorites, and the breads they are served on need not be unhealthy.

calories

Don't let terms like "hearty" fool you. Some hamburger and hot dog buns are high in calories, so check the label. They should be 120 calories or less per bun.

fiber

Fiber content is key. The best buns will have 2 grams of fiber or more per bun and little sugar.

healthiest choices

100% whole-wheat or white whole-wheat hamburger and hot dog buns are the healthiest choices out there.

sandwich rolls

Delicious and healthy sandwich rolls can make a good sandwich great.

calories

Stick with rolls that are 220 calories or less per roll.

fiber

Sandwich rolls should have at least 4 grams of fiber per roll.

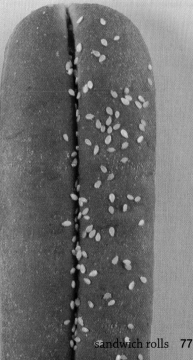

Watch out for portion size.

The main thing to look out for with sandwich rolls is the portion size. Extra-large rolls are often packed with calories. Follow the calorie guideline at left to help you decide which rolls are the best choice.

English muffins

These small, cornmeal-dusted muffins come in a variety of flavors, including some lower-calorie versions that are packed with fiber.

calories
Each muffin should contain 130 calories or less.

fiber
Each muffin should have at least 3 grams of fiber.

benefits
While similar in fat, iron, and sodium, 100% whole-wheat English muffins offer more zinc, magnesium, and vitamin E than their refined counterparts.

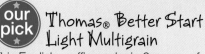

our pick — Thomas® Better Start Light Multigrain
This English muffin packs in 8 grams of healthy fiber for just 100 calories.

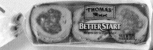

bakery muffins

Those huge muffins you see in the glass cases of bakeries and coffee shops may be giving you more than you bargained for.

calories
A bakery muffin should have 200 calories or less per serving. Typically these are the smaller 3-inch muffins.

fiber
Each muffin should have 2 grams of fiber or more.

🚩 Watch out for portion size.
Giant muffins, which often have added sugars and fat, can contain anywhere from 300 to 600 calories. While some are made with bran or blueberries, which offer a few more nutritional benefits over sugary doughnuts, the extra calorie load certainly isn't worth it.

believe it or not...

Although some supersized bakery muffins sound good for you, they're often not much healthier than a doughnut. You shouldn't eat the doughnut that often, either.

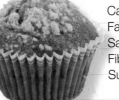

Calories: 470
Fat: 24 grams
Saturated fat: 8 grams
Fiber: 2 grams
Sugar: 32 grams

Calories: 200
Fat: 12 grams
Saturated fat: 6 grams
Fiber: less than 1 gram
Sugar: 10 grams

pitas

The healthiest pitas are 100% whole wheat, but look for other varieties that are made with whole grains and are high in fiber.

calories

- A 6-inch pita should contain 170 calories or less.
- A smaller 4-inch pita should have 75 calories or less.

fiber

- A 6-inch pita should contain at least 4 grams of fiber.
- A smaller 4-inch pita should have 2 grams of fiber or more.

wraps & flatbreads

Wraps and flatbreads make delicious alternatives to the typical sandwich bread.

calories
Whole-grain varieties should have 110 calories or less per wrap or flatbread.

fiber
There are a variety of brands that are packed with fiber. Look for ones with at least 5 grams per serving.

Arnold® Multigrain or 100% Whole-Wheat Sandwich Thins

Another option that's similar to flatbread is the sandwich thin. This circular roll is the perfect size for a burger or sandwich. It contains only 100 calories and has 5 grams of fiber per sandwich thin.

sliced breads

The variety of sliced breads in the grocery store is extensive. Here, we've highlighted the healthiest choices.

top 3 healthiest choices

100% whole wheat

calories
Each slice should contain 70 calories or less.

fiber
Each slice should have 2 grams of fiber or more.

benefits
This bread contains more protein and fiber than white bread for the same amount of calories.

white whole wheat

calories
Each slice should contain 70 calories or less.

fiber
Each slice should have 2 grams of fiber or more.

benefits
White whole-wheat bread looks and tastes like white bread but has the same nutritional benefits as regular whole-wheat bread. White whole wheat is made with an albino variety of wheat, which is the reason it more closely resembles white bread.

sprouted

calories
Each slice should contain 90 calories or less.

fiber
Each slice should have 2 grams of fiber or more.

benefits
The nutritional content of bread changes when the grain sprouts, so it's higher in protein, fiber, and certain vitamins and minerals. You'll find it in the freezer section.

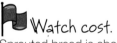 Watch cost.
Sprouted bread is about twice as expensive as regular bread.

You'll find some breads, often labeled "double fiber," that are loaded with fiber—5 grams or more per slice. This added fiber is from commercially produced isolated fibers, such as inulin or maltodextrin. While these isolated fibers increase the fiber count on the Nutrition Facts label and also provide bulk, they are structurally different from the intact fibers in whole foods, and they don't lower cholesterol or blood sugar. They're fine to eat, but it's best to turn to 100% whole grains to meet your fiber needs.

sliced breads, continued

rye

calories
Each slice should contain 80 calories or less.

fiber
Each slice should have 2 grams of fiber or more.

benefits
Pure rye bread contains only rye flour, which, unlike refined wheat flour, retains many of its nutrients during the milling process. Like oats, rye can help lower cholesterol. It's also a good source of fiber, magnesium, and protein. Some rye breads are made with a combination of rye and wheat flours, which is also a healthy choice.

light breads

calories
Each slice should contain 45 calories or less.

fiber
Each slice should have 1 gram of fiber or more.

benefits
There are a variety of light breads available in grocery stores. Lower-calorie bread is particularly helpful for those trying to lose or maintain weight.

fyi — light breads
Light breads usually have about half the calories of regular sliced bread. They are lightened by replacing some of the fat and flour with extra air and fiber.

fyi bakery bread

Grocery stores often offer freshly baked sliced breads filled with healthy ingredients like seeds, raisins, flax, oats, and millet that offer good-for-you fats, antioxidants, and added fiber. These items do add more calories, but if you're choosing breads made with whole grains, the benefits of these healthy additions can outweigh the extra calories. Stick with varieties that have fewer than 110 calories per slice and contain 3 grams of fiber or more.

Q&A What about other sliced breads?

The variety of sliced breads available is virtually endless as bread companies continuously offer new variations while different grocery stores and bakeries make their own. No matter what type of sliced bread you're buying, look to the ingredient list, calories, and fiber to guide your decision. Watch for healthy ingredients and select a bread that has 110 calories or less and 2 grams of fiber or more per slice.

tortillas

With so many tortillas on grocery store shelves, how do you know which to choose? Here's what you need to know to pick the healthiest ones.

flour tortillas

calories

For a 6-inch tortilla, 90 calories or less is ideal. For an 8-inch tortilla, look for those that have 130 calories or less. A 10-inch tortilla should have 180 calories or less.

fiber

Look for tortillas with at least 2 grams of fiber in a 6-inch size, 3 grams in an 8-inch size, and 5 grams in a 10-inch size.

benefits

Tortillas are another way to get a serving or two of whole grains. For flour tortillas, look for ones labeled "whole wheat." They contain iron and other B vitamins.

corn tortillas

calories

Each 6-inch corn tortilla should contain 75 calories or less.

fiber

Each 6-inch corn tortilla should have at least 1 gram of fiber.

benefits

To make sure you're getting some whole grains in your corn tortillas, select a brand that has "whole-grain corn" or "whole-grain cornmeal" listed first in the ingredient list. Corn tortillas are often made with minimal salt and very little added fat. One standard 6-inch tortilla contains only 42 milligrams of sodium and 1 gram of fat.

Watch out for extra-large portion sizes.
Calories can quickly add up as the size of the tortilla increases, so stick with those that are 10 inches or less.

Q&A Which tortilla is healthier?

A standard 6-inch corn tortilla contains about half the fat and calories and one-fourth the sodium of a similar-sized flour tortilla. In traditional Mexican tortillas, the fat comes from lard, but many brands now use vegetable shortening. Look for those made without trans fat.

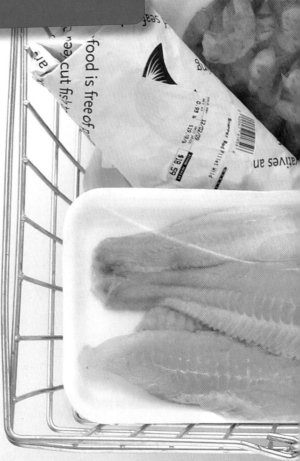

seafood

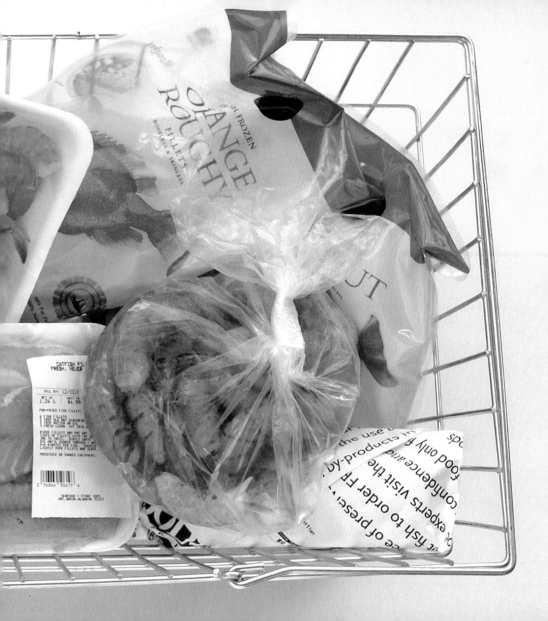

seafood

Why eat seafood?

Fish and shellfish contain:

- ☑ high-quality protein
- ☑ healthy unsaturated fats (particularly omega-3s)
- ☑ few, if any, saturated fats

How much should I eat?

Although the USDA's Dietary Guidelines don't make specific recommendations regarding seafood, other public health organizations, such as the American Heart Association and the American Dietetic Association, recommend two servings per week.

What is a serving?

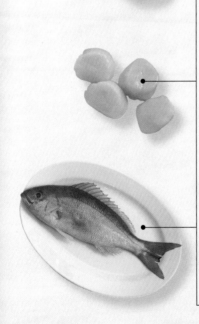

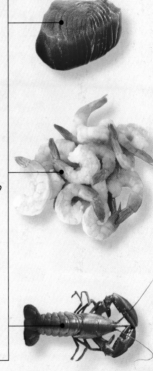

8-ounce bone-in fish steak (raw) = 1 serving

6-ounce fish fillet (raw) = 1 serving

6 ounces scallops (raw) = 1 serving

6 ounces peeled shrimp (raw) = 1 serving

12 ounces whole fish (raw) = 1 serving

1 (2-pound) lobster = 1⅓ servings

choose the healthiest seafood

With all of the press that seafood has received over the years, it's no wonder consumers are confused. Here's what you need to know.

1. Aim for variety.

The best approach when buying and eating seafood is variety. You'll consume varying levels of omega-3s from a number of sources without too much dependence on one. When shopping for seafood, let freshness be your guide. It's easy to substitute one fish for another, so if the mahimahi looks and smells fresher than the pompano, buy it instead.

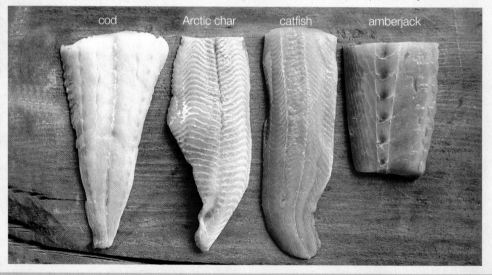

cod   Arctic char   catfish   amberjack

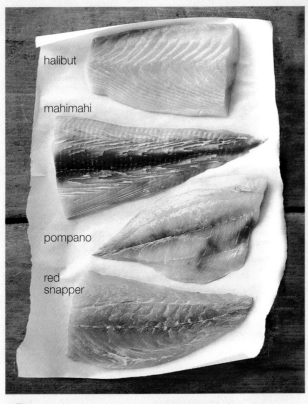

halibut

mahimahi

pompano

red
snapper

3. If you're concerned about sustainability, look for the logo.

The blue Certified Sustainable Seafood logo lets you know that the fish or shellfish you're buying is a sustainable choice. This logo was developed by the Marine Stewardship Council, which promotes sustainable fisheries and responsible fishing practices internationally, and it's only awarded to fisheries that meet strict environmental standards. Look for it on package labels, in grocery stores and shops that sell seafood, and in restaurants. But this seal isn't necessarily on all sustainable products, so do your homework on the sustainable seafood available in your area.

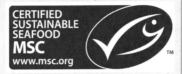

2. Buy in season.

Fish and shellfish have certain seasons when they are freshest, easiest to find, and the cheapest to buy. Check your local grocery stores to see what's in season in your area.

4. Eat seafood containing omega-3s a couple times per week.

Omega-3s are healthful polyunsaturated fats that help improve cardiovascular health by controlling cholesterol and reducing blood pressure. They're found in all types of fish and shellfish but are especially high in fatty fish. In general, shellfish and white-fleshed fish, such as cod, tilapia, and flounder, are low in all types of fat, including omega-3s, but that doesn't mean they should be avoided. They do provide a healthy source of lean protein.

seafood

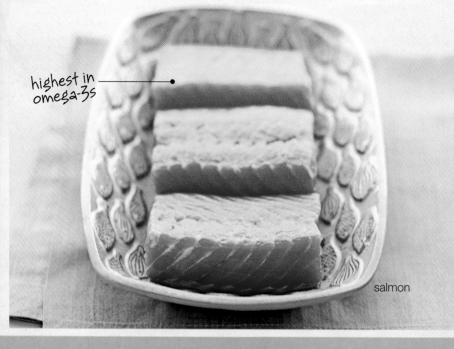

highest in omega-3s

salmon

How many omega-3s does your seafood have?

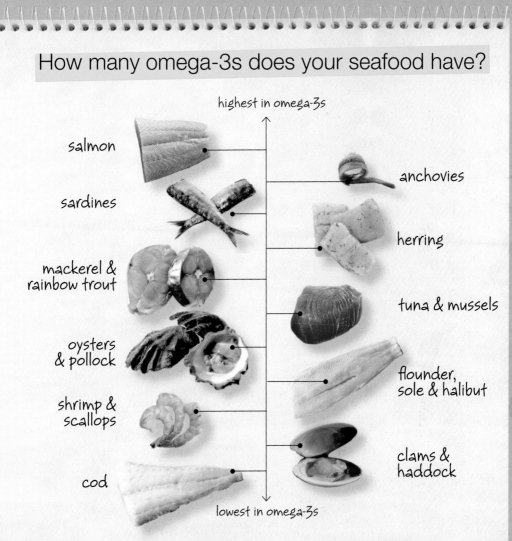

highest in omega-3s

salmon

anchovies

sardines

herring

mackerel & rainbow trout

tuna & mussels

oysters & pollock

flounder, sole & halibut

shrimp & scallops

clams & haddock

cod

lowest in omega-3s

source: USDA Nutrient Database for Standard Reference

95

watch out for these red flags

For the most part, seafood is good for you, but there are a few things to be mindful of.

🚩 Watch out for seafood from the same local source.

For those who buy seafood caught in a nearby lake, bay, or river, it's important to be aware of the potential contaminants in that water source (such as runoff from farms or sewage treatment plants). If you regularly consume seafood from that same source, your exposure levels to a particular contaminant in the water will be higher than if you eat from a variety of sources. Check with your local or state environmental health department for the current warnings.

Watch out for mercury.

Some fish and shellfish contain high levels of mercury that can inhibit brain development in fetuses and young children. As a result, the Food and Drug Administration and the Environmental Protection Agency often issue seafood safety advisories for pregnant women, women who may become pregnant, nursing mothers, and young children, encouraging them to avoid some types of fish and shellfish and to eat only seafood with lower levels of mercury. Those with the highest levels of mercury include shark, swordfish, king mackerel, and tilefish. Check local advisories about the safety of fish and shellfish caught in local lakes, rivers, bays, and coastal areas.

Watch out for seafood labeled organic.

There currently isn't a USDA-approved organic label for seafood, although it certainly isn't for lack of trying. The complications arise because it's difficult to apply and regulate land-based agriculture standards to seafood, particularly wild seafood in open waters. However, some states do allow seafood labeled as organic from other countries. But be aware that there's no way to guarantee those products are indeed organic.

fish

With so many choices available, where do you start when choosing fish? Here are some helpful tips.

seafood

In 16 of the 20 countries with the lowest rates of heart disease, people consumed significantly higher quantities of fish.

fish nutrition

Fish is an excellent source of high-quality protein that is also low in cholesterol. And it's generally a good source of B vitamins, especially niacin, B_{12}, and B_6.

medium and dark-fleshed fish

These types of fish, such as salmon and tuna, are generally higher in fat, including heart-healthy omega-3 fatty acids (see page 95), and are good sources of vitamins A and D. Some, such as fresh sardines and smelt, contain small, soft, edible bones, which are valuable sources of calcium.

white-fleshed fish

In general, white-fleshed fish, such as cod, tilapia, flounder, and grouper, are low in all types of fat, including healthful omega-3s. But these choices are excellent sources of lean protein and shouldn't be avoided.

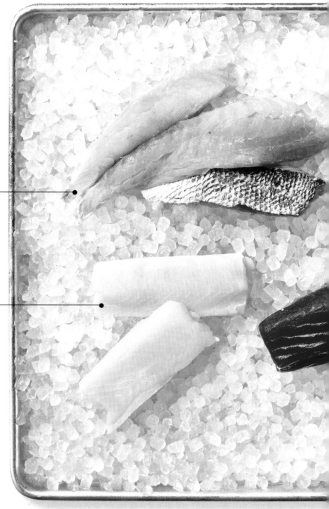

types of fish

Fish can be categorized many ways, but we've created five groups based on color and fat content.

white, lean & flaky

- Black sea bass
- Flounder
- Rainbow smelt
- Red snapper ————————
- Tilapia

white, firm & oil rich

- Albacore tuna
- Atlantic shad
- California white sea bass
- Chilean sea bass ————————
- Cobia
- Lake trout
- Lake whitefish
- Pacific escolar
- Pacific sablefish
- Trout (rainbow)
- Weakfish (sea trout)
- White sturgeon
- Whiting

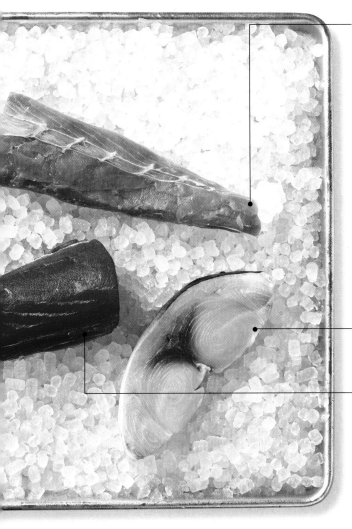

medium color & oil rich

- Amberjack
- Arctic char
- Mahimahi
- Paddlefish
- Pompano
- Salmon (Coho)
- Salmon (sockeye)
- Yellowfin tuna

white, lean & firm

- Alaska pollock
- Catfish
- Grouper
- Haddock
- Pacific cod
- Pacific halibut
- Pacific rockfish
- Pacific sand dab and sole
- Striped bass (wild and hybrid)
- Swordfish

dark & oil rich

- Anchovies
- Bluefin tuna
- Herring
- Mackerel (Atlantic or Boston)
- Mackerel (king)
- Salmon (Chinook or king)
- Salmon (farmed)
- Sardines
- Skipjack tuna

fish, continued

believe it or not...

In a study published by the *Journal of the American Medical Association*, scientists calculated that if 100,000 people ate farmed salmon twice a week for 70 years, the extra PCBs (polychlorinated biphenyls) could potentially cause 24 extra deaths from cancer, but the omega-3s consumed would prevent at least 7,000 deaths from heart disease.

Q&A Should I eat wild or farmed salmon?

The debate between the two is based on the levels each contains of potentially cancer-causing PCBs (polychlorinated biphenyls). Farmed salmon is generally higher in PCBs, which is why it's often placed on do-not-buy lists. However, the levels found in these fish are still generally very low, and most health experts agree that the benefits of salmon's omega-3s outweigh the risk posed by PCBs. Plus, farmed salmon is widely available and reasonably priced.

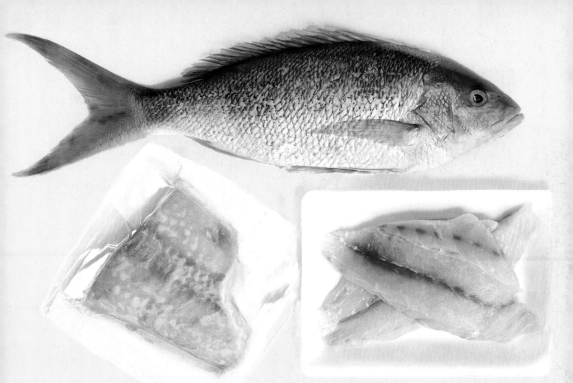

fresh vs. frozen

Nutritionally, fresh and frozen fish are the same. Unless you live near water, it can be challenging to find fresh fish. Often the "fresh" fish you buy from the fish counter has been previously frozen. For top quality, look for "frozen-at-sea" (FAS)—fish that has been flash-frozen at extremely low temperatures in as little as three seconds onboard the ship. When thawed, frozen-at-sea fish is virtually indistinguishable from fresh.

shellfish

Shellfish come in many packages, but all are rich in protein and low in calories and saturated fat.

shellfish nutrition

clams

Clams are rich in selenium, phosphorus, and iron—6 ounces contain your daily iron needs.

crabs

Crabs offer vitamin B12, selenium, and phosphorus, and they're also rich in calcium and folate. A 6-ounce portion contains 15% of your daily calcium needs and almost 19% for folate.

crawfish

Crawfish is a good source of folate and phosphorus.

lobster

Lobster is an excellent source of phosphorus and also provides a dose of calcium.

mussels

Mussels are low in sodium and cholesterol and contain omega-3 fatty acids. They're also a good source of folate—a 6-ounce portion contains almost 18% of your daily needs.

oysters

Oysters are packed with minerals such as zinc and selenium as well as omega-3s. They also contain a healthy portion of your daily iron needs. A 6-ounce serving contains 100% of the daily iron requirement for men and almost 75% for women.

shrimp & scallops

Both offer about a day's worth of vitamin B12 and are rich in selenium and phosphorus. Shrimp offers about eight times as much iron as scallops (nearly one-fourth of a woman's daily needs), while scallops pack in five times more folate per serving.

fyi scallop packaging

"Wet packed" scallops have been treated with a liquid solution containing sodium tripolyphosphate. The scallops absorb this mixture and plump up, resulting in a heavier weight and a higher market price. But when you cook them, the liquid portion will cook out, leaving you with smaller scallops and a higher sodium content. "Dry packed" scallops are not chemically treated and are preferable over wet packed for price and lower sodium content.

shellfish, continued

imitation crab

Imitation crab, also labeled crab sticks, usually does not contain much, if any, crab. It's actually a processed seafood made from surimi, a white fish that has been ground into a paste and mixed with flavor concentrate made from crab, shrimp, scallops, or lobster. In the United States, most imitation crab meat is made from Alaskan pollock. Whiting is also sometimes used, but its flesh is so soft that egg white and potatoes have to be added for the mixture to be firm enough for processing.

Imitation crab is usually lower in cholesterol than real crab but higher in sodium.

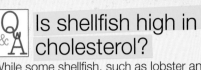

Is shellfish high in cholesterol?

While some shellfish, such as lobster and shrimp, are high in cholesterol, that doesn't mean you shouldn't eat them. Cholesterol found in food has little effect on blood cholesterol in most people. It's really the saturated fats and trans fats in foods that are the most important factors affecting blood cholesterol levels. Both fats are known to increase total cholesterol, including the bad stuff—LDL cholesterol.

meats &
poultry

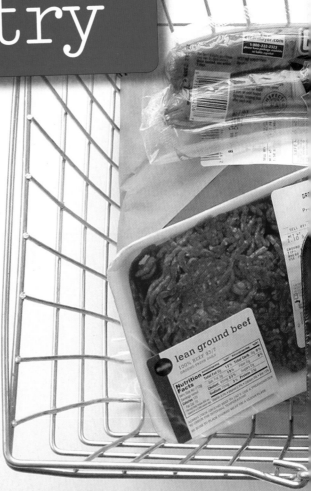

lean ground beef

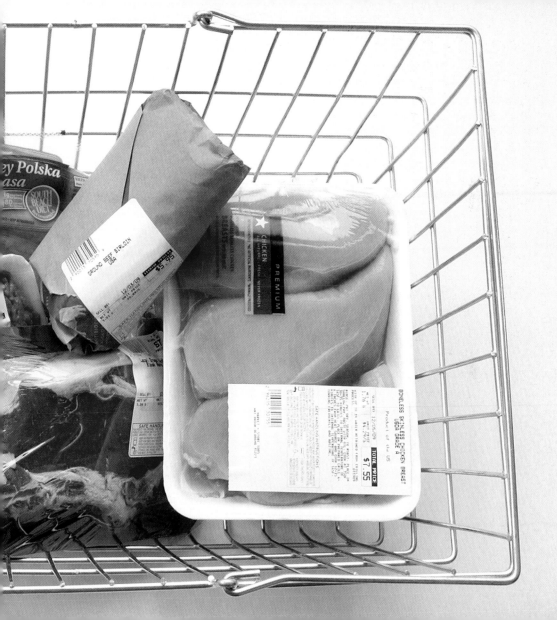

meats & poultry

Why eat meats and poultry?

Meat and poultry contain:
- ☑ protein
- ☑ iron
- ☑ B12
- ☑ zinc
- ☑ phosphorus

This is the amount of protein the average person needs daily.

How much should I eat?

The USDA doesn't provide specific recommendations for meats and poultry. Instead, it gives a protein recommendation, which you can fulfill from meats, poultry, seafood, eggs, nuts, seeds, peas, and beans. While the specific amount of protein you need depends on your age, gender, and level of physical activity, most adults need about 1 to 1½ servings (the equivalent of 5 to 6½ ounces of cooked protein or about 30 to 45 grams of protein) per day. For healthy adults, consuming more protein in a day shouldn't be a health concern.

What is a serving?

1 (6-ounce) chicken breast (raw) = 1 serving

1 (4-ounce) boneless pork loin chop (raw) = $\frac{2}{3}$ serving

1 (4-ounce) beef tenderloin steak (raw) = about $\frac{2}{3}$ serving

1 (4-ounce) boneless lamb chop (raw) = about $\frac{1}{2}$ serving

1 (4-ounce) boneless veal chop (raw) = $\frac{1}{2}$ serving

1 ($\frac{1}{4}$-pound) burger patty (raw) = about $\frac{2}{3}$ serving

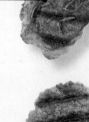

choose the healthiest meats & poultry

Although meats and poultry may contain saturated fat and cholesterol, they can still be part of a healthy diet. Here's how:

1. Choose lean cuts.

There are many choices available in the grocery store when it comes to meats and poultry, so it's important to know which cuts are the healthiest. You'll find information about the leanest cuts of meat and the best poultry choices on the following pages.

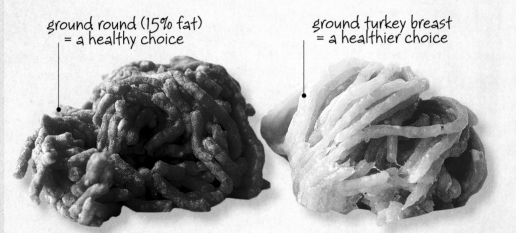

ground round (15% fat)
= a healthy choice

ground turkey breast
= a healthier choice

2. Trim away excess fat and remove the skin.

Trimming visible fat and removing the skin on meats and poultry will help lower total fat, saturated fat, and calories. Simply removing the skin from a chicken breast reduces the calories by 42% and the fat by 88%.

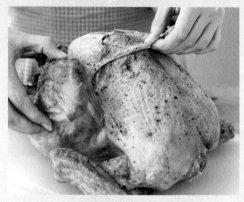

3. Practice portion control.

In general, Americans have no problem meeting their protein requirements. And while excess protein may not be harmful to you if you're in good health, it's the excess saturated fat and calories that often come along with it that can lead to problems. Use the serving size guidelines (page 111) and our recommendations throughout this chapter to guide you.

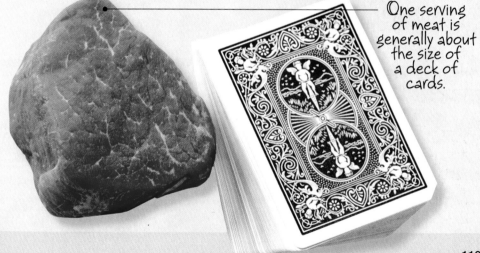

One serving of meat is generally about the size of a deck of cards.

watch out for
these red flags

Meat and poultry contain many healthful nutrients, but there are some things to keep an eye on.

Watch out for processed meats.

It's best to limit your intake of processed meats, such as sausage, bologna, salami, and hot dogs. Many processed meats, including those labeled "reduced fat" or "⅔-less-fat," are still high in saturated fat, calories, and sodium. Read the labels carefully to make sure you know what you're buying.

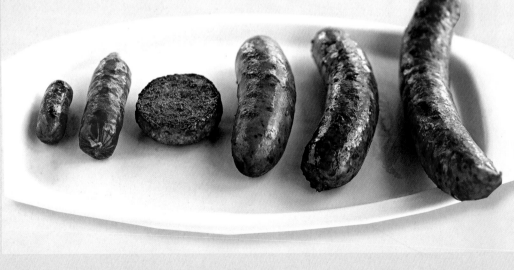

⚑ Watch out for meat with lots of marbling.

Marbling is the intramuscular fat found in meat, especially red meat. It adds juiciness and flavor, but it also adds saturated fat. Since you can't remove this fat, the easiest way to avoid it is by choosing leaner meats.

⚑ Watch out for saturated fat.

High saturated fat content is a primary concern, especially with red meat. Saturated fat raises your LDL cholesterol and can lead to heart disease by encouraging the formation of plaque in the arteries. Choose leaner cuts so you'll benefit from all the vitamins, minerals, and high-quality protein that meats offer without the unhealthy saturated fats.

Meats high in saturated fat tend to have a lot of marbling.

BEEF SKIRT STEAK(OUTSIDE SKIRT)
(USDA INSPECTED)

Product of the US and Canada,
Mexico

SELL BY: 01/21/09	TOTAL PRICE
NET WT 0.37 lb UNIT PRICE $8.99/lb	$3.33

MARINATE IN TENDERIZING MARINADE (SALSA,
ITALIAN DRESSING, ETC) 6-24 HOURS. GRILL,
UNCOVERED OVER MED ASH-COVERED COALS, FOR
MED RARE TO MED DONENESS. GRILL 17-21 MIN
FOR 1 1/2 TO 2 LB STEAK, TURNING ONCE.
OR BROIL ON RACK OF BROILER PAN SO SURFACE
OF BEEF IS 2-3" FROM HEAT, FOR MED RARE TO
MED DONENESS. BROIL 13-18 MIN FOR 1 1/2 TO
2 LB STEAK, TURNING ONCE.

SAFE HANDLING INSTRUCTIONS

THIS PRODUCT WAS PREPARED FROM INSPECTED AND PASSED MEAT AND/OR POULTRY. SOME FOOD
PRODUCTS MAY CONTAIN BACTERIA THAT COULD CAUSE ILLNESS IF THE PRODUCT IS MISHANDLED
OR COOKED IMPROPERLY. FOR YOUR PROTECTION, FOLLOW THESE SAFE HANDLING INSTRUCTIONS.

☐ KEEP REFRIGERATED OR FROZEN
☐ THAW IN REFRIGERATOR OR MICROWAVE   ☐ COOK THOROUGHLY
☐ KEEP RAW MEAT AND POULTRY SEPARATE
   FROM OTHER FOODS. WASH WORKING SURFACES
   (INCLUDING CUTTING BOARDS), UTENSILS, AND
   HANDS AFTER TOUCHING RAW MEAT OR POULTRY.   ☐ KEEP HOT FOODS HOT
                                                 REFRIGERATE LEFTOVERS
                                                 IMMEDIATELY OR DISCARD

beef

Beef can be a healthy choice. The key is choosing lean cuts so you aren't buying more saturated fat and calories than you bargained for.

For the healthiest beef, buy "choice" or "select" grades rather than "prime." Prime cuts aren't as lean.

lean cuts

Select lean cuts of meat with minimal visible fat. In addition to flank steak, tenderloin, loin, sirloin, chuck shoulder, and arm roasts, try the lean cuts listed on page 117.

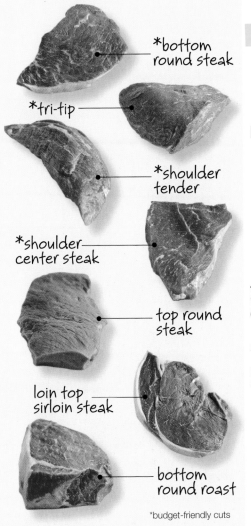

*bottom round steak

*tri-tip

*shoulder tender

*shoulder center steak

top round steak

loin top sirloin steak

bottom round roast

*budget-friendly cuts

ground beef

Look at the percentages to guide you when buying ground beef. If the package is labeled "80% lean," that means it's 20% fat. In addition to ground chuck (20% fat), round (15% fat), and sirloin (10% fat), you may also find ground beef simply labeled "lean ground beef." At 7% fat, it's the leanest ground beef available. If the package just says "ground beef" that's an indication that it contains more than 20% fat.

ground round (15% fat)

our pick

*ground sirloin (10% fat)

lean ground beef (7% or less fat)

*What *Cooking Light* most frequently uses in recipes calling for ground beef.

beef 117

beef, continued

making sense of the beef label

"grain-fed/grain-finished beef"

Most U.S. beef comes from cattle fattened on grain, usually corn. Since corn is not part of a cow's natural diet, the animal may experience stress and illness, so they're routinely treated with antibiotics. They also typically receive growth hormones, which cause them to gain weight faster.

"grass-fed/grass-finished beef"

This beef comes from cattle that forage on grass and legumes. It's lower in saturated fat, cholesterol, and calories than grain-finished beef.

⚑ Watch out for cost.

Raising grass-finished cattle is time-consuming and requires large open spaces, which contribute to the higher price tag.

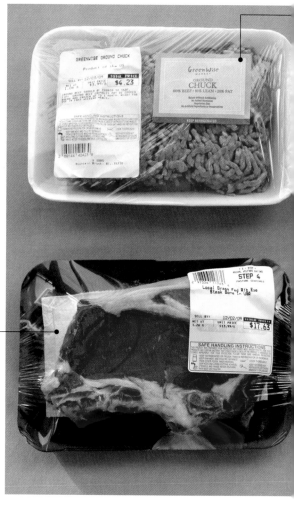

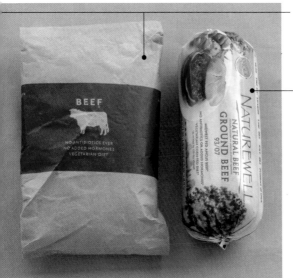

"no hormones or antibiotics added"

This means that the animals were raised without hormones or antibiotics.

"natural"

Beef labeled "natural" must not contain any artificial ingredients and cannot be more than minimally processed, as ground beef is. The label must explain their use of the term, such as "no added colorings or artificial ingredients" or "minimally processed." The difference between natural and organic beef is the feed. Though naturally raised livestock are usually fed a vegetarian diet, the feed may have been grown using pesticides.

 Do I need to buy organic meat? USDA ORGANIC

Meat from conventionally raised animals causes concern because of the synthetic hormones given to the animals to quickly increase their weight. The side effects are still being investigated, but they could potentially disrupt hormone balance and cause developmental problems and a variety of cancers. Animals raised organically are not given hormones or antibiotics, are fed 100% organically, and must be fed on pasture for at least 120 days each year. All organic meat in the U.S. will have the USDA-certified organic label on the package.

veal & lamb

These young, tender cuts of meat offer a lean source of protein, but they come at a higher price than some other meats.

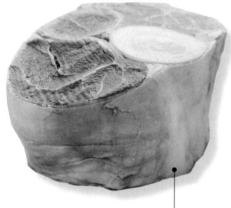

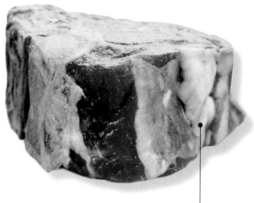

lean cuts

veal

The leanest cuts are the leg cutlet, arm steak, sirloin, rib chop, loin chop, and top round. You can also purchase ground veal, which is generally very lean.

lamb

For the leanest cuts of lamb, look for "loin" or "leg" on the label. Some lean cuts include the leg loin, chops, arm chops, and foreshanks. Ground lamb is also fairly lean and can be used in the same way as ground beef.

🚩 Watch out for cost.

The reason for the higher price tag is simply that these meats require more attention and nurturing to produce such tender cuts.

pork

This "other white meat" is indeed packed with protein, and many cuts are low in fat.

lean cuts

The leanest pork choices include tenderloin, boneless top loin chops, boneless top loin roast, center loin chops, center rib chops, and bone-in sirloin roast.

making sense of the pork label

"no hormones added"

Hormones are not allowed to be used when raising hogs. Therefore, this claim can't be used on pork labels unless it's followed by the statement: "Federal regulations prohibit the use of hormones."

"natural"

Pork labeled "natural" must not contain any artificial ingredients and cannot be more than minimally processed, as ground pork is. The label must explain their use of the term, such as "no added colorings or artificial ingredients" or "minimally processed."

"no antibiotics"

The animals were raised without the use of antibiotics. Antibiotic use is a growing public health concern because it may contribute to human antibiotic resistance.

ground pork

For the healthiest choice, select ground pork that's labeled "lean ground pork." Pound for pound, it contains less fat and calories than ground sirloin, which has 10% fat.

pork, continued

ham

The primary concern with ham is its sodium content. Choose varieties labeled "less-sodium" as a healthier option.

sausage

Pork sausage can be high in saturated fat, calories, and sodium. Look for a lower-fat version—there are 50%-less-fat varieties available—or try lean turkey sausage. Check the label for sodium and choose the one with the lowest amount per serving.

bacon

Bacon is fatty—it's a concentrated source of saturated fat and sodium, but that doesn't mean you have to eliminate it from your diet. Use less of the full-fat variety, or, for a healthier choice, choose center-cut bacon. It has the same satisfying flavor, but because it's cut closer to the bone, it contains about 20% less saturated fat than regular bacon. A serving of two slices of center-cut bacon is modest in calories (40 calories) and saturated fat (1 gram), plus the sodium is reasonable (173 milligrams).

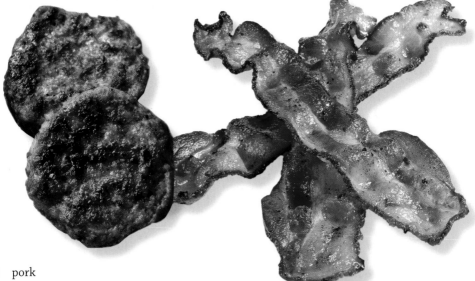

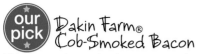

our pick — Dakin Farm® Cob-Smoked Bacon

This bacon is smoked over corncobs, which gives it sweetness and a more subtle smokiness than its wood-smoked cousins. A bonus is that this brand had the second-lowest sodium level of all bacons tested, with just 93 milligrams per slice—even less than some of the lower-sodium bacons.

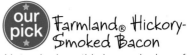

our pick — Farmland® Hickory-Smoked Bacon

Not only does this bacon look perfect (it doesn't curl when cooked, and it turns an even golden brown), but it also has a great balance of sweet, salty, and smoky flavors that makes it a great all-purpose bacon.

best overall

good choice

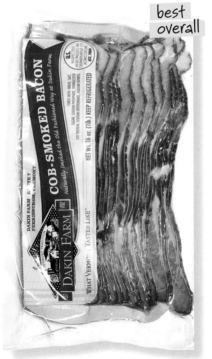

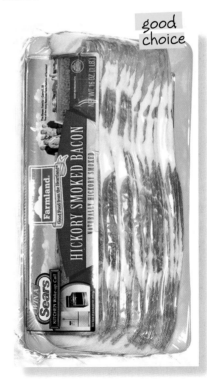

poultry

Both chicken and turkey are traditional favorites. They're lean, flavorful, readily available, and relatively inexpensive.

lean cuts

Within poultry, there are two types of meat: the light meat and the dark meat. The healthier of the two is the light meat, which includes the breast, since it contains less saturated fat (about 50% less) than the dark thigh, leg, and wing meat. The dark meat is dark simply because those muscles are used more and have more myoglobin proteins. In nonflying birds like turkey and chicken, the legs become dark while the breast meat stays light.

fyi   duck & goose

In flying birds, like duck and geese, their whole bodies contain dark meat, which means they're higher in saturated fat. For everyday meals using poultry, stick with chicken and turkey breast meat, and reserve flying birds for special occasions.

dark meat:
4 ounces has 3g
of saturated fat

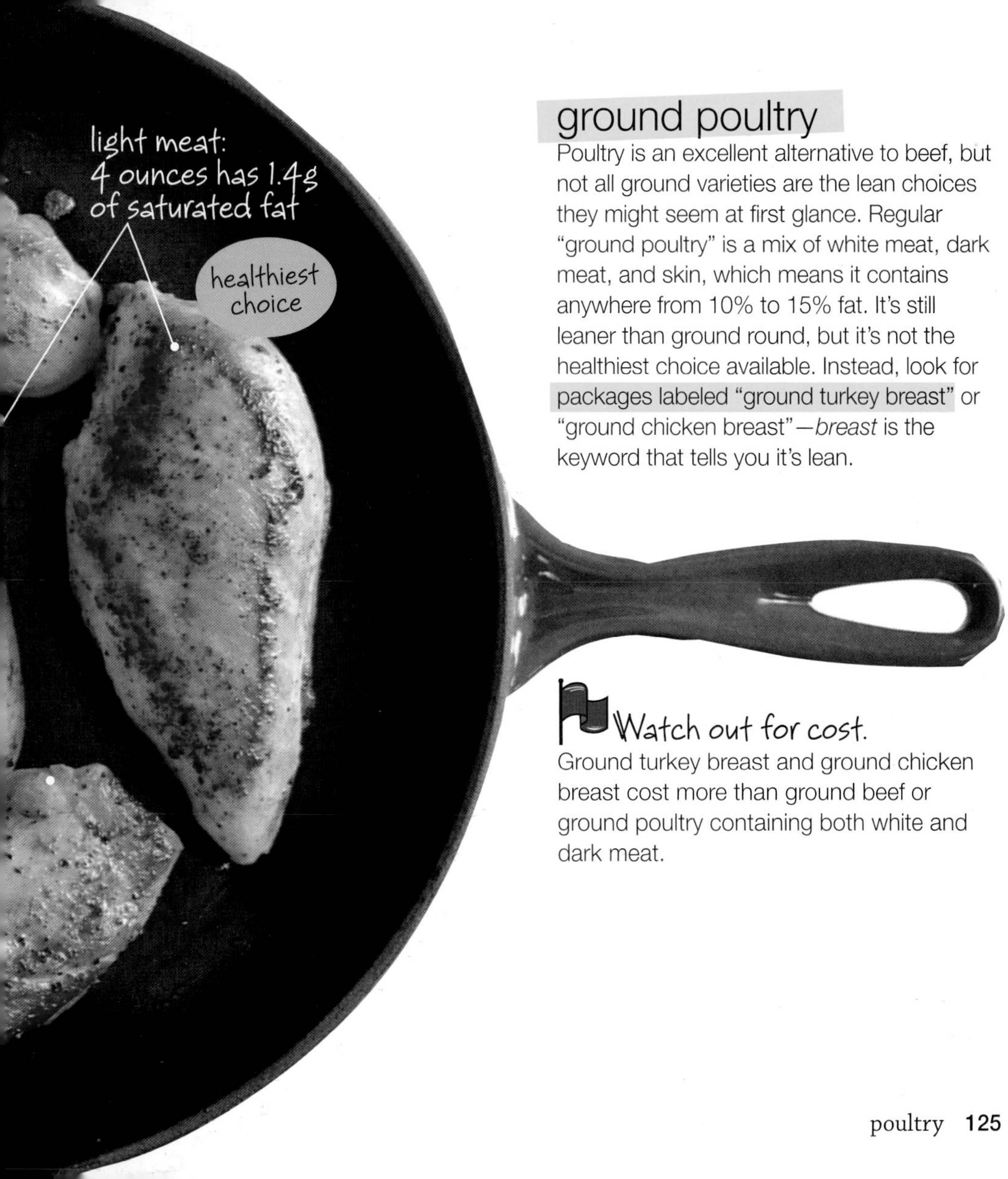

light meat:
4 ounces has 1.4g
of saturated fat

healthiest
choice

ground poultry

Poultry is an excellent alternative to beef, but not all ground varieties are the lean choices they might seem at first glance. Regular "ground poultry" is a mix of white meat, dark meat, and skin, which means it contains anywhere from 10% to 15% fat. It's still leaner than ground round, but it's not the healthiest choice available. Instead, look for packages labeled "ground turkey breast" or "ground chicken breast"—*breast* is the keyword that tells you it's lean.

Watch out for cost.

Ground turkey breast and ground chicken breast cost more than ground beef or ground poultry containing both white and dark meat.

poultry, continued

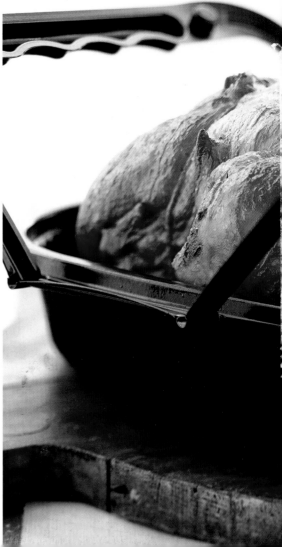

making sense of the poultry label

"free range" or "free roaming"

The animals have been allowed to go outside.

"no hormones added"

Hormones are not allowed to be used when raising poultry. Therefore, this claim can't be used on poultry labels unless it's followed by the statement: "Federal regulations prohibit the use of hormones."

"no antibiotics"

The animals were raised without the use of antibiotics. Antibiotic use is a growing public health concern because it may contribute to human antibiotic resistance.

"natural"

Poultry labeled "natural" must not contain any artificial ingredients and cannot be more than minimally processed, as ground poultry is. The label must explain their use of the term, such as "no added colorings or artificial ingredients" or "minimally processed."

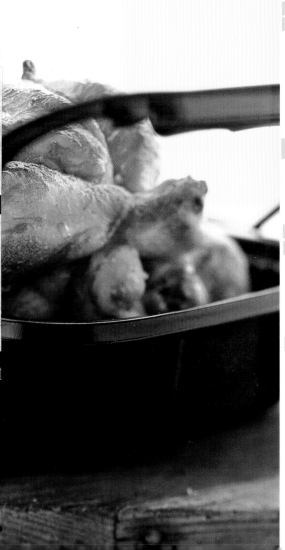

rotisserie chicken

Rotisserie chickens are a convenient and healthy choice when the skin is removed. They're available in a variety of flavors, and all are great options, since most of the added sodium will be discarded with the skin. And, as always, the light meat is better for you than the dark meat.

bacon & sausage

turkey bacon

When compared to regular pork bacon, turkey bacon offers fewer calories and less fat. However, its nutritional profile is similar to that of center-cut pork bacon, so take your pick of those two healthier options.

turkey & chicken sausage

Turkey and chicken sausage are both lower in fat and calories than traditional sausage, but the real savings is in saturated fat—they have nearly half.

Watch out for sodium.

Turkey and chicken sausage may be smoked and still be relatively high in sodium. Check the label and opt for the brand with the lowest amount of sodium per serving, and then watch your portion size.

deli-sliced meats

The high sodium content of convenient prepackaged and deli-sliced meats makes them a nutritional challenge.

lean cuts

Choose lean turkey, roast beef, ham, or low-fat deli meats. They're the healthiest options out there. Two to three ounces or less per sandwich or serving is really ideal. You can always have the deli slice it thin so your three ounces stack higher.

Watch out for high-fat meats.

Bologna and salami are some of the worst deli offenders. They contain about 65% more calories and 88% more saturated fat per serving that their leaner counterparts mentioned above.

Watch out for sodium.

No matter how you slice it, it can be hard to find a prepackaged or sliced deli meat that doesn't have a high amount of sodium. Some of these meats, including typical deli ham, are cured in salt, which increases the sodium content. There are a variety of lower-sodium meats out there, some of which contain half the sodium of regular deli meat, so opt for those when possible. If a lower-sodium variety isn't available, read the nutrition label to find the one with the lowest amount of sodium per serving—ideally less than 350mg of sodium per 2-ounce serving. Always watch your portion size. It's easy to pile on an extra slice or two, but you may be piling on more than you think.

meats & poultry

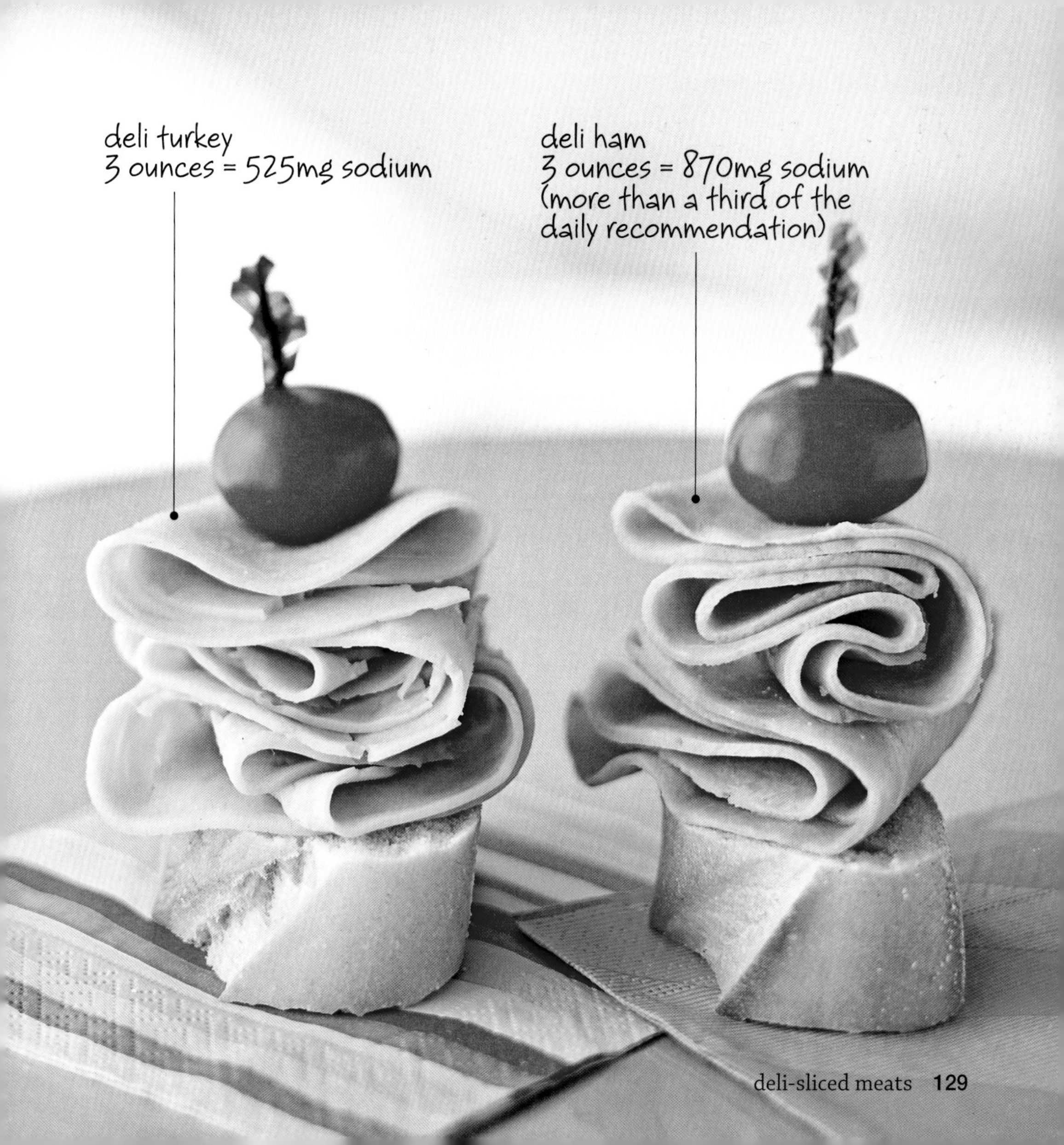

deli turkey
3 ounces = 525mg sodium

deli ham
3 ounces = 870mg sodium
(more than a third of the
daily recommendation)

dairy & eggs

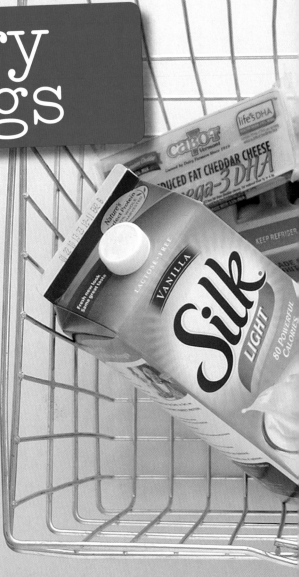

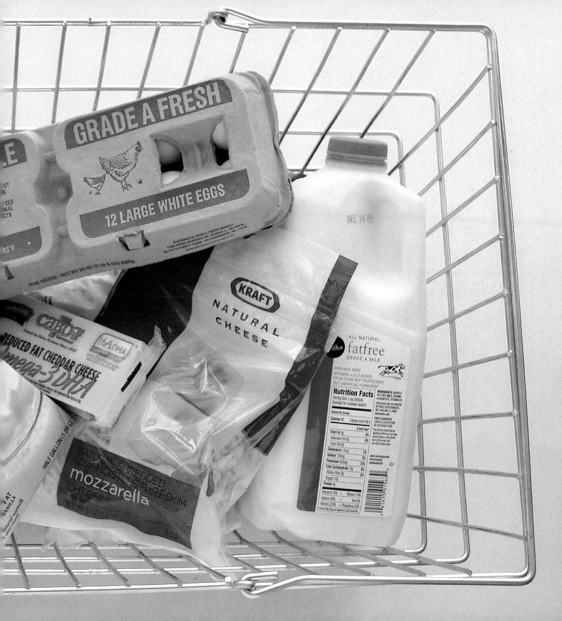

dairy & eggs

Why eat dairy?

Milk and other dairy products contain:

- ☑ calcium
- ☑ vitamin D
- ☑ protein
- ☑ vitamin B12
- ☑ vitamin A
- ☑ phosphorus

Why eat eggs?

Eggs contain:

- ☑ protein
- ☑ iron
- ☑ vitamin B12
- ☑ folate

How much should I eat?

For dairy, the USDA's Dietary Guidelines recommend that adults should consume 3 servings of milk or other dairy products per day, particularly low-fat or fat-free products. Children ages 2 to 8 should consume 2 servings per day. For eggs, there is no specific recommendation, but they can count towards your daily protein requirement of 1 to 1½ servings per day (about 30 to 45 grams of protein). One egg has 6.3 grams of protein.

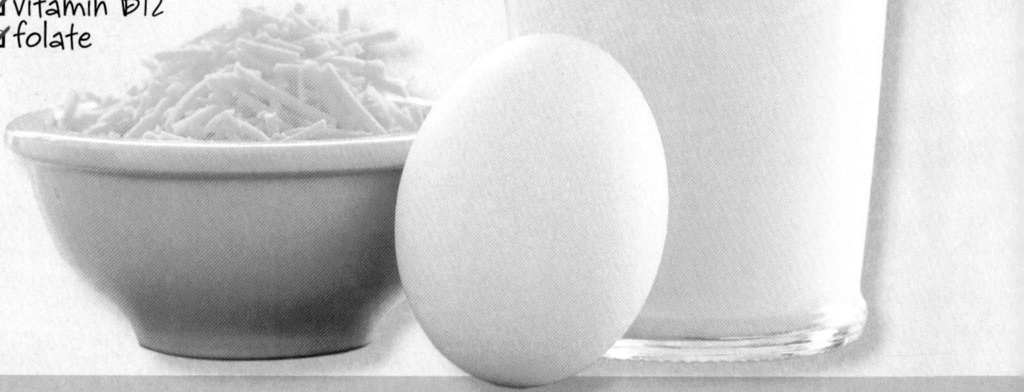

What is a serving?

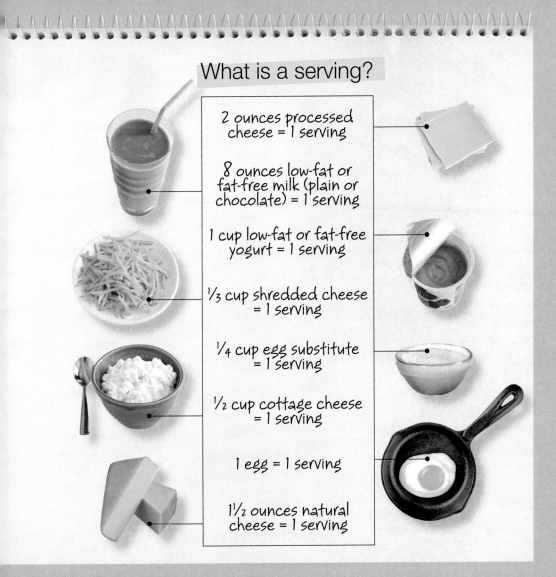

2 ounces processed cheese = 1 serving

8 ounces low-fat or fat-free milk (plain or chocolate) = 1 serving

1 cup low-fat or fat-free yogurt = 1 serving

1/3 cup shredded cheese = 1 serving

1/4 cup egg substitute = 1 serving

1/2 cup cottage cheese = 1 serving

1 egg = 1 serving

1 1/2 ounces natural cheese = 1 serving

choose the healthiest dairy & eggs

Supermarket shelves are stocked with an assortment of dairy products and egg choices. Here you'll learn how to make the most of them.

1. Enjoy cheese in moderation.
While cheese provides health benefits—it's a good source of protein and is rich in calcium—it is a nutrient-dense food that comes with saturated fat and sodium. Ounce for ounce, cheese contains about six times the amount of saturated fat than that found in beef tenderloin, and on average, a 1-ounce slice of cheese contains about 10% of your daily sodium allotment. By all means, eat cheese, but do so in moderation.

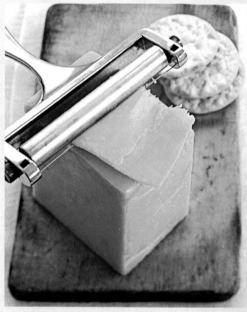

2. Choose fat-free or low-fat dairy products.

Most major health organizations, including the USDA in their Dietary Guidelines for Americans, recommend you choose low-fat or fat-free milk and other dairy foods to meet the recommended daily servings. We agree; low-fat or fat-free milk is ideal for everyday applications, like drinking or pouring over cereal. However, all forms of dairy find a place in our diets, depending on need. Check out the following pages for the details.

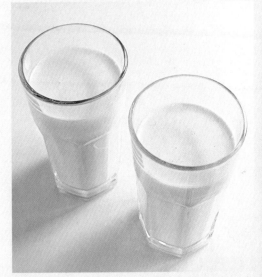

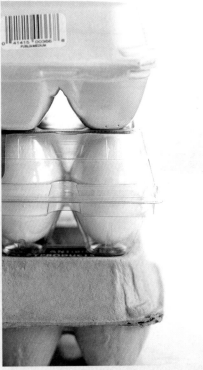

3. Eggs really are pretty incredible.

One egg has 13 essential nutrients, including high-quality protein, folate, iron, and zinc, all in a compact 70-calorie package. See page 153 to learn more.

watch out for these red flags

Even with all the health attributes found in dairy and eggs, there are still a few things to keep in mind.

Watch out for raw milk.
The dairy industry, the FDA, and the Centers for Disease Control and Prevention strongly support pasteurization for safety reasons. Milk contains bacteria that, when handled improperly, may multiply. However, demand for raw milk is growing, and in some states, consumers can buy raw milk and cheese with certain restrictions. Advocates believe that raw milk is healthier and tastier and that pasteurization destroys beneficial bacteria, proteins, and enzymes. However, because of these bacteria, it's important for pregnant women, children, the elderly, and the immune-compromised to avoid raw milk and products that are made from it.

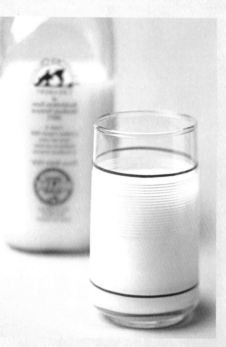

🚩 Watch out for lactose intolerance.

A high proportion of adults from non–Northern European backgrounds are lactose intolerant, which means they can't digest lactose, the primary sugar found in milk. To better tolerate lactose, introduce foods slowly, drink lactose-free milk (shown at right), choose aged cheeses that are low in lactose, or take the enzyme lactase to help digestion.

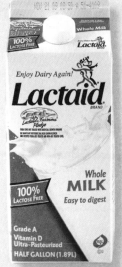

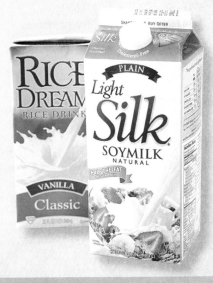

🚩 Watch out for nondairy sources of calcium that aren't fortified.

While it's certainly possible to get calcium from nondairy sources, such as soy milk, be sure to read the label carefully to make sure the product you're buying is fortified with calcium.

milk

For most everyday applications, fat-free milk is ideal, but other milks have their place in a healthy diet. Here's what you need to know.

selecting the best

fat-free (skim) milk
Per cup: 83 calories, 0.2g fat (0.1g sat fat)
Best uses: Due to its low calorie and fat content, this milk is the everyday ideal—as a drink, on cereal, in oatmeal. It also contains the most calcium per serving.

1% (low-fat) milk
Per cup: 102 calories, 2.4g fat (1.5g sat fat)
Best uses: This is a good second choice behind fat-free milk, since it's still relatively low in calories.

2% (reduced-fat) milk
Per cup: 122 calories, 4.8g fat (3g sat fat)
Best uses: This is a better alternative than whole for everyday use, but it's still not as good as 1% or fat-free milk.

whole milk
Per cup: 146 calories, 8g fat (4.5g sat fat)
Best uses: Children under 2 need to drink whole milk, but adults and older children should go for a lower-fat or fat-free milk.

half-and-half
Per cup: 315 calories, 28g fat (17g sat fat)
Best uses: Using this in small doses, such as in a cup of coffee, is OK. The fat-free version is a healthier choice for more regular use.

heavy cream
Per cup: 821 calories, 88g fat (55g sat fat)
Best uses: The fat and calorie content of this dairy product means it should be an occasional treat.

fyi dairy alternatives

For those who don't eat dairy, choose calcium-fortified alternative milk made from rice, soy, hemp, oats, or almonds. All are lactose and cholesterol free and low in fat. Shake well before drinking; the valuable calcium sinks to the bottom of the cartons.

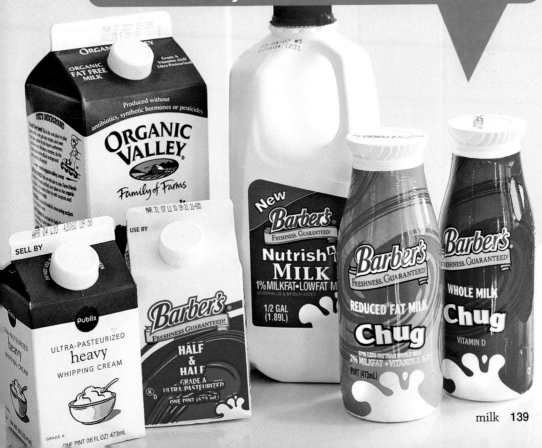

Moove to a more healthful milk. Do it in steps. If you use half-and-half in your coffee, switch to whole milk. From whole, go to 2% milk. Then try 1% or fat-free milk.

milk **139**

milk, continued

healthiest choice

less fat, more calcium

Because calcium is contained in the nonfat part of milk, reduced-fat dairy foods contain slightly more of the mineral than full-fat varieties. Below is the amount of calcium in milligrams found in an 8-ounce serving of each type of milk.

Whole	2%	1%	Fat free
276 mg	285 mg	290 mg	306 mg

buttermilk

Despite its name, buttermilk doesn't contain butter. It's "cultured," meaning it's created by fermenting pasteurized fat-free or low-fat milk with a friendly bacteria culture in the same way that yogurt and sour cream are made. Opt for fat-free (or nonfat) buttermilk. It contains 40% fewer calories and 0 grams of saturated fat, compared to the 5 grams found in regular buttermilk.

soy milk vs. cow's milk

fyi

Both plant-based soy milk and cow's milk offer roughly equal amounts of protein. If you buy soy milk, make sure you're choosing one that's fortified. If not, you're only getting a fraction of the calcium found in cow's milk.

dairy & eggs

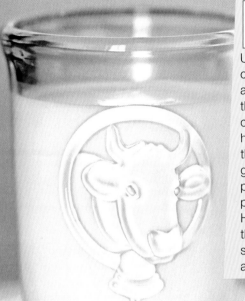

Q&A Should I buy organic milk?

USDA rules require that organic cows be fed on organic pasture for at least 120 days out of the year so they can obtain plenty of fresh grass. Organic cows also cannot be treated with synthetic hormones. All cows generate natural hormones that help them produce milk, but some are given a synthetic version that boosts milk production by as much as one gallon a day per cow. According to the FDA, the World Health Organization, and others, milk from these cows is safe, but the use of this synthetic hormone is illegal in many countries, and critics question its safety.

yogurt

Yogurt is a creamy cultured milk with all the normal benefits of dairy—bone-strengthening calcium, heart-healthy potassium, and filling protein—plus a pleasant taste.

selecting the best

There are many nutritional benefits in yogurt: satiating protein plus calcium and other minerals that keep your bones, muscles, and tissues strong. Yogurt is concentrated milk, and milk contains about 12 grams of natural sugar (lactose) per cup. Choose low-fat or fat-free nonflavored yogurts to minimize saturated fat and added sugar. You may notice that some yogurts are high in fiber—some contain 5 grams per serving. This extra fiber isn't naturally found in yogurt; it comes from inulin, a commercially produced isolated fiber. While it provides bulk, it's structurally different from the intact fibers found in whole foods and doesn't lower cholesterol or blood sugar.

Watch out for high-sugar yogurts.

More than 25 grams of sugar per serving in a yogurt may mean added sugars, often in the form of jelly-like fruit on the bottom. Instead, customize your cup with fresh fruit or choose flavored varieties that aren't aimed at your sweet tooth.

Greek yogurt has more protein and less sodium than regular fat-free yogurt.

Greek vs. plain yogurt

Greek yogurt is strained to remove most of the whey or liquid, a process that makes it thicker. One serving contains 7 additional grams of protein and half the sodium of regular fat-free yogurt. But you'll find three times the calcium (about one-third of a day's recommended amount) in the regular variety. A cup of either counts as one of the three recommended daily servings of dairy.

Regular fat-free yogurt has three times more calcium than Greek yogurt.

yogurt, continued

plain yogurt

our pick

Chobani® Non-Fat Plain

This is the best plain yogurt we've found. Besides being loaded with 18 grams of satiating protein, this boasts the creamy thickness of Greek-style yogurt. This fat-free version keeps both calorie and saturated fat counts well within reasonable ranges.

yogurt drink

our pick

Lifeway® Organic Low-Fat Kefir

As our favorite yogurt drink, kefir (of Turkish origin, meaning "good feeling") technically is a cultured milk drink, not a yogurt. But it has similar flavor and a nutritional edge over other yogurt drinks: more protein and vitamin D with less sugar.

flavored yogurt

our pick

Stonyfield Farm® Organic Low-Fat Blueberry

This is our favorite flavored yogurt. Organic milk is the first ingredient; blueberries are the second. What's not to love? Other flavors are similarly simple. This has a modest amount of sugar plus bone-strengthening vitamin D.

probiotics

Probiotics are live microorganisms, usually bacteria, that are similar to the healthy bacteria found in the human digestive tract. They yield a health benefit when eaten in proper amounts. Researchers are still studying which microorganisms perform best and how much of them we need, but preliminary studies indicate some types may reduce cavity-causing bacteria in the mouth, while others may boost immunity or digestive health. The challenge when grocery shopping can be figuring out if the yogurt you're buying contains probiotics, since there are no standard labeling requirements. Look for brands that have the scientific names of the specific probiotic strains used in the yogurt listed on the label and that offer consumers easy access to studies supporting their claims.

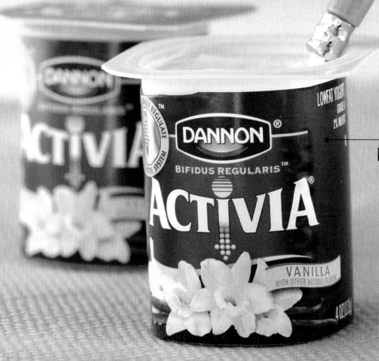

This yogurt contains the probiotic bifidus regularis, which may be good for your digestive tract.

cheese

Cheese is undeniably delicious, but it is also a nutrient-dense food. Follow these tips to help you make the best choice.

selecting the best

fat-free cheese
Per ¼ cup: 45 calories, 0g fat (0g sat fat)
Best uses: For weight loss, the low calorie content of this cheese is helpful. However, the taste and texture is quite different than even reduced-fat cheese, and it doesn't melt the same way regular cheese does.

reduced-fat cheese

our pick

Per ¼ cup: 86 calories, 6.5g fat (4.3g sat fat)
Best uses: This is a good all-around cheese option. It's healthier than whole-milk cheese, but it still has the pleasing taste and texture that make cheese worth eating. But with all cheese—reduced fat or otherwise—moderation is key.

whole-milk cheese
Per ¼ cup: 114 calories, 9.4g fat (6g sat fat)
Best uses: This cheese contains a lot of calories and saturated fat. Reserve it for special occasions.

Watch out for sodium.
Many cheeses can be high in sodium, so read the label to know exactly how much you're getting.

---

fyi Swiss cheese

Swiss is one variety of cheese that's naturally low in sodium—a 1-ounce slice contains 75mg of sodium compared to 175mg in a similarly sized slice of Cheddar.

There are so many varieties of cheese, and not all come in a lower-fat version. The best tip: Practice portion control and enjoy every bite.

ricotta cheese

Ricotta cheese is made from whey—the liquid that separates out from the curds when cheese is made. The variety made from whole milk is high in saturated fat (a ½-cup portion contains the majority of the daily recommendation), so follow the same guidelines you would when choosing milk, and select a fat-free or reduced-fat version. You'll save substantially on both saturated fat and calories.

cottage cheese

Cottage cheese is made from milk with varying levels of fat, so you'll see full-fat, 2%, 1%, and fat-free versions. The best choice is the fat-free variety, but 1% isn't a bad second choice, since it has the same amount of calories and only a marginal increase in saturated fat (0.7g in a ½ cup of 1% compared to zero in the fat free).

dairy & eggs

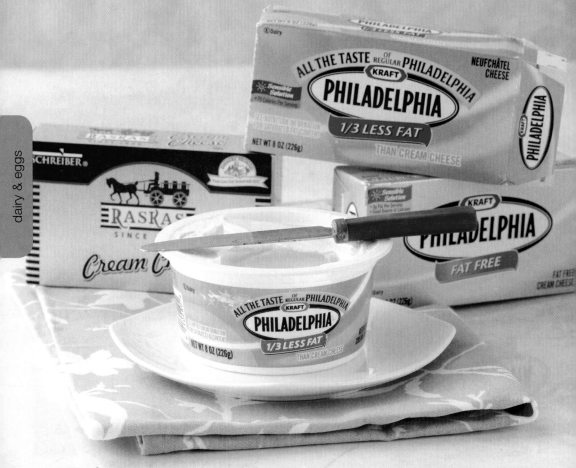

selecting the best

fat-free cream cheese

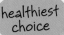
healthiest choice

Per tablespoon: 14 calories, 0.2g fat (0.1g sat fat)
Best uses: With its low saturated fat content, this cream cheese is a great choice for everyday use.

⅓-less-fat cream cheese

Per tablespoon: 36 calories, 3.1g fat (2.1g sat fat)
Best uses: This is a great middle-of-the-road option, although moderation is key, since one tablespoon contains about 13% of the daily recommendation for saturated fat. You might also see this labeled as Neufchâtel.

whole-milk cream cheese

Per tablespoon: 51 calories, 5.1g fat (3.2g sat fat)
Best uses: The full-fat version packs in a lot of calories and fat. Reserve it for special occasions.

Watch out for processed cheese.

The blocks of processed cheese—the ones that don't have to be refrigerated, last a long time, and are the basis of many popular cheese dips—are not *really* cheese. They're something known as "processed cheese," "cheese food," or "cheese product." While they are made from real cheese, they have additives that make them more shelf-stable and uniform in texture and color. The primary differences among these highly processed "cheeses" are found in their fat and moisture content and optional ingredients, such as flavorings, that may be added. If you do eat these, opt for the light versions available that are lower in fat and sodium.

butter

There is simply no substitute for butter. Although made up completely of fat, butter can still have a small spot in a healthy diet.

selecting the best

stick butter

Per tablespoon: 100 calories, 11g fat (7.2g sat fat)
Best uses: In moderation, stick butter is the best choice for baking.

cultured cream butter

Per tablespoon: 100 calories, 11g fat (7g sat fat)
Best uses: Made by adding lactic acid to butter; some people prefer its sharper taste. Can be used in any application that calls for butter.

yogurt-based butter

Per tablespoon: 45 calories, 5g fat (1g sat fat)
Best uses: This is a great choice for everyday use, since it contains significantly fewer calories and saturated fat than regular butter. It's not suitable for baking.

whipped butter

Per tablespoon: 68 calories, 7.7g fat (4.8g sat fat)
Best uses: This is a good choice to serve at the table because it's spreadable even when cold.

European-style butter

Per tablespoon: 100 calories, 11g fat (7g sat fat)
Best uses: Because of its lower water content, this type of butter has a rich flavor. You can use it in any application for which you would use butter.

light butter

Per tablespoon: 65 calories, 7.2g fat (4.5g sat fat)
Best uses: This butter has half the fat and calories of regular butter. It's fine as a spread, but its lower fat content makes it a poor choice for baking or frying.

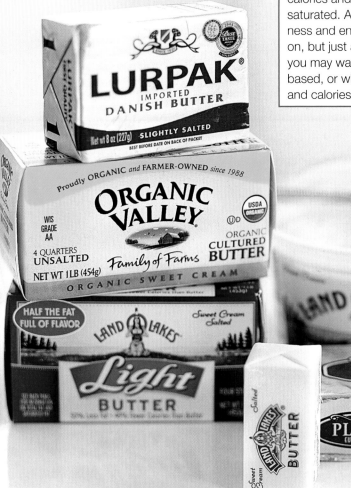

Q & A What should I buy—butter or margarine?

It depends. Margarine has often been thought of as more beneficial for heart health, since it's made from vegetable oils and is higher in good mono- and polyunsaturated fats, while butter is made from animal fats and contains more saturated fat and cholesterol. However, not all margarines are created equal and some may even be worse than butter. Most margarines are processed using a method called hydrogenation, which creates unhealthy trans fats, and in general, the more solid the margarine, the more trans fats it contains (making stick margarine worse than tub). When buying margarine, select one with the lowest trans-fat content possible (ideally, one that has 0 grams and doesn't list "partially hydrogenated oils" in the ingredient list) and the lowest amount of saturated fat (ideally, less than 2 grams). Or, instead of margarine, choose another one of the healthier butter options listed on page 150. If you use butter, use it in moderation.

fyi heart-healthy spreads

You'll find some buttery spreads out there geared specifically to heart health. They're made with a blend of vegetable oils that can help improve your cholesterol ratio. These spreads are also free of the hydrogenated oils that create unhealthy trans fats. Be aware, these better-for-you alternatives also carry a higher price tag.

eggs

Budget-friendly and packed with protein, eggs are a great nutritional package. Simply open and use.

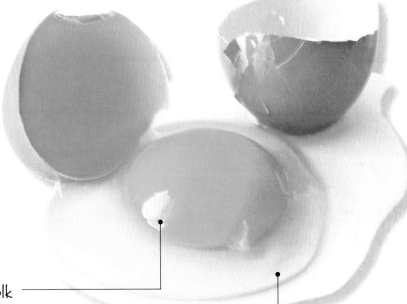

the yolk

The yolk contains all of an egg's fat and any fatty acids (such as omega-3s), about half the protein, most of the vitamins (such as A, B_{12}, and E), and all of the antioxidants. Because it contains all the fat, it contains 76% of an egg's calories.

the white

The white accounts for more than half of an egg's protein and minerals, such as iron, selenium, and trace amounts of calcium.

eggs, continued

egg labels, unscrambled

USDA Organic

To meet the standards of the USDA's National Organic Program, birds must be cage free, fed on organic pasture for at least 120 days each year, fed organic vegetarian food, and cannot be given antibiotics.

United Egg Producers Certified

This certification attests that a company gives food and water to its caged hens. The following terms are unregulated, and therefore have no meaning: natural, naturally raised, no hormones, no antibiotics.

Animal Welfare Approved

A new label by the Animal Welfare Institute is given to independent family farmers with flocks of up to 500 birds, where chickens are free to spend as much time as they desire outside on pesticide-free pasture, cannot have their beaks trimmed (a practice often done in crowded egg farms), and cannot be fed animal by-products. Since this label applies to smaller egg producers, you may only find it at farmers' markets or specialty grocers.

Certified Humane Raised & Handled

A program audited by the USDA and endorsed by many animal welfare organizations with humane requirements for raising and handling chickens and their eggs.

Cage Free

The chickens are out of cages with continuous access to food and water but may not necessarily have access to the outdoors.

sizing up eggs

Egg sizes cause the nutrition profile to vary slightly.
Cooking Light usually uses large eggs.

Small	Medium	Large	Extra Large	Jumbo
54 cal	63 cal	72 cal	80 cal	90 cal
3.8g fat	4.4g fat	5g fat	5.6g fat	6.3g fat
1.2g sat fat	1.4g sat fat	1.6g sat fat	1.7g sat fat	2g sat fat

Q&A What's in those egg substitutes?

Egg substitutes are basically egg whites with a bit of food coloring added. Some brands may also contain added flavorings like spices, salt, or onion powder. Because it's the egg whites, egg substitutes contain half the calories of eggs and don't contain any fat and cholesterol. However, they lack many of the nutrients found in yolks, including iron, vitamins D and B12, and riboflavin. One-fourth of a cup of egg substitute is equal to one large egg.

fyi

eggs & cholesterol

Eggs do have a place in a heart-healthy diet. For years, the high cholesterol content of eggs placed them on the list of bad-for-you foods, but a large Harvard School of Public Health study found no association between eating up to one egg a day and heart disease, except in people with diabetes.

condiments, dips & oils

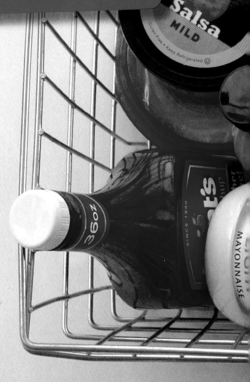

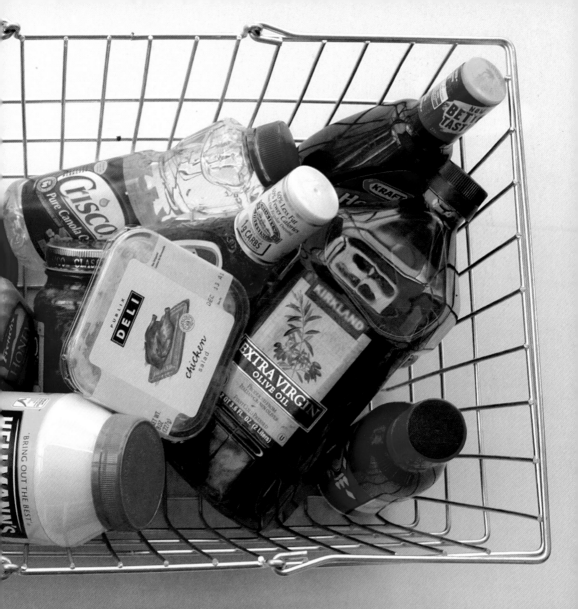

condiments, dips & oils

Why eat condiments, dips, and oils?

Condiments and dips add flavor, and depending on what you choose, they can contribute valuable nutrients, too, such as:

- ☑ healthy fats
- ☑ antioxidants
- ☑ vitamins
- ☑ minerals

Oils contain:

- ☑ healthy mono- and polyunsaturated fats
- ☑ vitamin E

How much should I eat?

The USDA doesn't provide specific guidelines for condiments. However, most condiments fall into the discretionary calories category—each person has a very small daily allowance (between 100 and 300 calories). Go to MyPyramid.gov to determine your needs. The guidelines for prepared salads or dips depends on the ingredients used to make them. For those that are produce-based, the guidelines for fruits and vegetables would apply (see page 30); for meat-based salads, those daily guidelines would apply (see page 110).

The USDA suggests daily allowances for oils, since they can be a source of healthful fats. For adults, these vary from 5 to 7 teaspoons daily based on age, gender, and activity level. Foods that naturally contain oil, such as nuts, and foods that are mainly oil, such as oil-based salad dressings, count.

What is a serving?

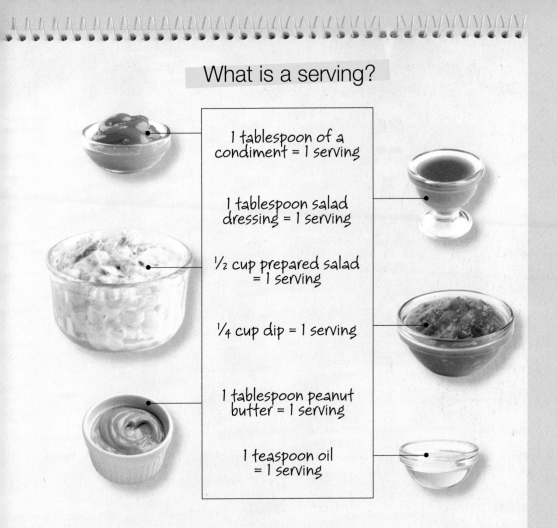

1 tablespoon of a condiment = 1 serving

1 tablespoon salad dressing = 1 serving

½ cup prepared salad = 1 serving

¼ cup dip = 1 serving

1 tablespoon peanut butter = 1 serving

1 teaspoon oil = 1 serving

choose the healthiest condiments, dips & oils

Condiments, dips, and oils can enhance bland, boring meals by adding much-needed flavor. And if you choose wisely, these flavor boosters can also add healthy nutrients.

1. Choose oils with the least amount of saturated fats.
Saturated fats are an unhealthy type of fat that can increase your risk for heart disease by increasing your total cholesterol, including your "bad" LDL cholesterol. When choosing oils, look for those with a higher percentage of mono- and polyunsaturated fats. These fats, if used in place of saturated fats, can lower your risk of heart disease.

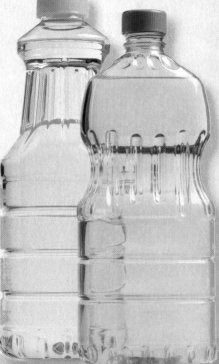

2. Choose plant-based dips.

Fruit, vegetable, bean, and legume-based dips flavored with spices and herbs are the healthiest options because they pack in vitamins, minerals, antioxidants, and filling fiber.

> For everyday snacking, choose lower-calorie options like salsa or hummus.

3. Choose low-calorie condiments and dips for everyday use.

Let's face it—there are some condiments and dips that are just naturally high in fat. By all means, enjoy them, but do so in moderation and only on occasion. For everyday meals, choose lower-calorie options that add flavor without breaking the nutritional bank. Use the guidelines throughout this chapter to help you choose.

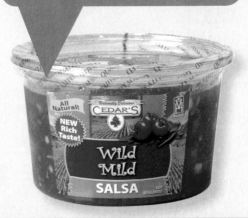

watch out for these red flags

These extra additions to your meal can bring more to the table than just added flavor.

🚩 **Watch out for creamy, full-fat condiments and dips.**
Rich sauces and dips can pack in an ample number of calories and saturated fat. It's best to select light, reduced-fat, or fat-free varieties. If the full-fat version is all that's available, practice portion control and pay close attention to the nutrition label so you know exactly what you're getting.

Pay attention to portion size when adding creamy condiments to your sandwiches, salads, and meals.

162

Watch out for prepared salads.

Prepared salads may be convenient, but they aren't usually doing you many nutritional favors. While the ingredients are often listed on the label, the Nutrition Facts label isn't always there, so there's no way to really know what you're getting. In these cases, use our guidelines on page 178 to help you make the healthiest selection. The best choice, however, is usually to make your own so you can control what goes in them.

Watch out for sodium.

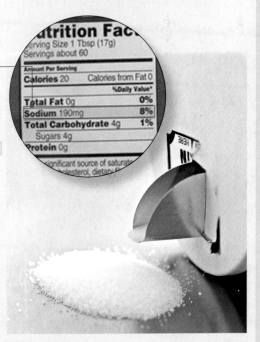

Americans have no problem meeting (and often exceeding) their daily sodium recommendation of 2,300 milligrams. That excess sodium often comes from takeout, processed, and prepared foods, as well as extras like condiments. Be sure to check the label of all condiments, even those that you don't think will contain a high amount of sodium, and always watch your portion size. If there is a salt-free or reduced-sodium variety available, choose that. But be aware that even these lower-sodium versions can contain a relatively high amount of sodium per serving, so be careful how much you add.

condiments

These tasty additions can add lots of flavor and, depending on the kind you select, some nutritional benefits.

ketchup and mustard

Mustard is the condiment of choice for calorie counters, though ketchup has a nutritional edge. A tablespoon of mustard has fewer calories and no sugar. But the same amount of ketchup provides more than twice the potassium, plus lycopene, a phytochemical found in tomatoes that may help prevent heart disease and some cancers. In fact, lycopene is more concentrated in processed tomato products than in fresh varieties. Ketchup also contains a number of carotenoids, such as beta-carotene; these pigments found in bright-colored fruits and vegetables may help ward off cancer.

specialty mustards

Mustards are an excellent low-calorie, low-saturated fat option for adding tons of flavor. Any of these are a great choice—just watch the sodium.

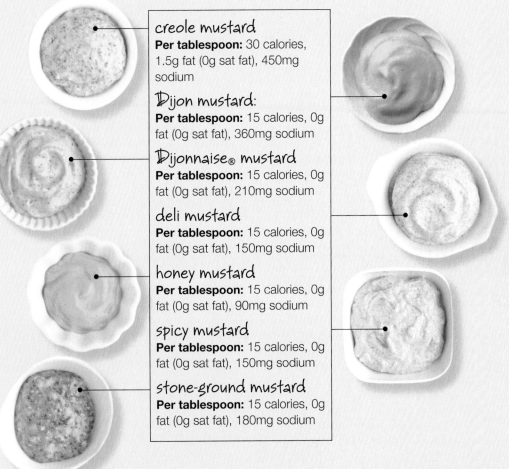

creole mustard
Per tablespoon: 30 calories, 1.5g fat (0g sat fat), 450mg sodium

Dijon mustard:
Per tablespoon: 15 calories, 0g fat (0g sat fat), 360mg sodium

Dijonnaise® mustard
Per tablespoon: 15 calories, 0g fat (0g sat fat), 210mg sodium

deli mustard
Per tablespoon: 15 calories, 0g fat (0g sat fat), 150mg sodium

honey mustard
Per tablespoon: 15 calories, 0g fat (0g sat fat), 90mg sodium

spicy mustard
Per tablespoon: 15 calories, 0g fat (0g sat fat), 150mg sodium

stone-ground mustard
Per tablespoon: 15 calories, 0g fat (0g sat fat), 180mg sodium

condiments, continued

mayonnaise

real mayonnaise
Per tablespoon: 90 calories, 10g fat (1.5g sat fat)
Best uses: It's best to only use this high-calorie mayo on occasion.

light mayonnaise
Per tablespoon: 35 calories, 3.5g fat (0g sat fat)
Best uses: A good option for everyday use. But if you're watching your calorie intake closely, go with the reduced-fat or low-fat mayo, and choose the one that tastes the best to you.

reduced-fat mayonnaise
Per tablespoon: 20 calories, 2g fat (0g sat fat)
Best uses: A good option for everyday use.

low-fat mayonnaise
Per tablespoon: 15 calories, 1g fat (0g sat fat)
Best uses: A good option for everyday use.

condiments, dips & oils

fyi | tartar sauce

This condiment can be calorie-heavy depending on the type you select—in fact, 1 tablespoon of the full-fat version can contain 80 calories and 1.5 grams of saturated fat. Choose a light, reduced-fat, or low-fat variety to save on both calories and saturated fat.

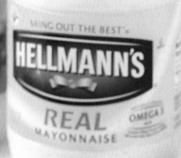

mayonnaise made with canola oil

Per tablespoon: 45 calories, 4.5g fat (0g sat fat)

Best uses: This is a great all-around mayonnaise option. While the fat content may be 4.5 grams per tablespoon, it's the heart-healthy unsaturated kind.

mayonnaise made with olive oil:

Per tablespoon: 50 calories, 5g fat (0.5g sat fat)

Best uses: A good option for everyday use, since most of its fat comes from healthy unsaturated fats.

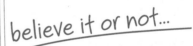

believe it or not...

Despite its reputation, mayonnaise alone doesn't cause foodborne illness. It's made of acidic ingredients (vinegar, lemon juice, and salt) and heat-treated pasteurized eggs that discourage bacterial growth. Problems arise when mayonnaise is mixed with contaminated foods, the mixture is stored improperly, or both.

condiments, continued

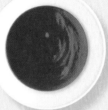

barbecue sauce

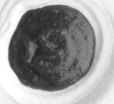

cocktail sauce

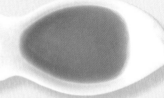

fish sauce

hoisin sauce

honey

horseradish

believe it or not...

If stored at room temperature in an airtight container, honey can remain good for decades or even centuries. Pots of honey discovered in ancient Egyptian tombs were found to still be edible after thousands of years. This is due to honey's low water content and relatively high acidic level, which discourages the growth of bacteria or other microorganisms.

other condiments

barbecue sauce

The thicker the barbecue sauce, the more calories it contains, so opt for a flavorful thinner sauce or choose one that has 30 calories or less per tablespoon.

Per tablespoon: 30 calories, 0g fat (0g sat fat), 120mg sodium

---

fyi **light BBQ sauce**

Generally, light barbecue sauces contain more water and vinegar and have fewer calories than their thicker counterparts.

---

cocktail sauce

This flavorful ketchup-based condiment offers a concentrated source of lycopene with minimal calories.

Per tablespoon: 15 calories, 0.1g fat (0g sat fat), 200mg sodium

fish sauce

Fish sauce contains very few calories and no fat, but this is a condiment to watch because it contains a lot of sodium. Use it sparingly.

Per tablespoon: 6 calories, 0g fat (0g sat fat), 1,200mg sodium

hoisin

This Chinese sauce, which is similar to barbecue sauce, is fragrant and pungent and adds a burst of salty-sweet flavor to a dish. Watch out for the sodium though. Different brands can contain widely different amounts of sodium, so be sure to select the brand that has the lowest amount per serving.

Per tablespoon: 45 calories, 1.5g fat (0.3g sat fat), 230mg sodium

honey

This natural ingredient is an excellent way to add sweetness to dishes.

Per tablespoon: 64 calories, 0g fat (0g sat fat), 1mg sodium

horseradish

This mixture of vinegar and the ground root of the horseradish plant is a healthy, flavorful, low-sodium option.

Per tablespoon: 7 calories, 0.1g fat (0g sat fat), 47mg sodium

condiments, continued

hot sauce

This spicy condiment certainly adds a kick to any dish, and it contributes minimal calories and sodium for the flavor boost.
Per tablespoon: 2 calories, 0.1g fat (0g sat fat), 89mg sodium

marinades

There are tons of different marinade options, and different brands have considerable nutritional differences. While there may be some variation in the calories per serving, the primary concern is sodium, which can range anywhere from 150mg to 900mg per tablespoon. When making your choice, look for a reduced-sodium variety.

soy sauce

While soy sauce may be skinny on calories, it's hefty on sodium. Be sure to select the "lite" version and use it sparingly.
Per tablespoon ("lite" version): 10 calories, 0g fat (0g sat fat), 605mg sodium

steak sauce

When using this with your steak (or any other meat), watch your portion size because those extra spoonfuls can quickly add up to lots of sodium at one sitting.
Per tablespoon: 15 calories, 0g fat (0g sat fat), 200mg sodium

syrup

Syrup is a calorie-dense food that's mostly sugar. Choose a "lite" syrup that contains about half the calories of regular.
Per tablespoon ("lite" version): 25 calories, 0g fat (0g sat fat), 45mg sodium

teriyaki sauce

Soy sauce is one of the main ingredients in this sweet-salty sauce, which means sodium is a concern. Select a "lite" teriyaki sauce and use it sparingly.
Per tablespoon ("lite" version): 19 calories, 0g fat (0g sat fat), 411mg sodium

Worcestershire sauce

This sauce has minimal calories and no fat.
Per tablespoon: 11 calories, 0g fat (0g sat fat), 167mg sodium

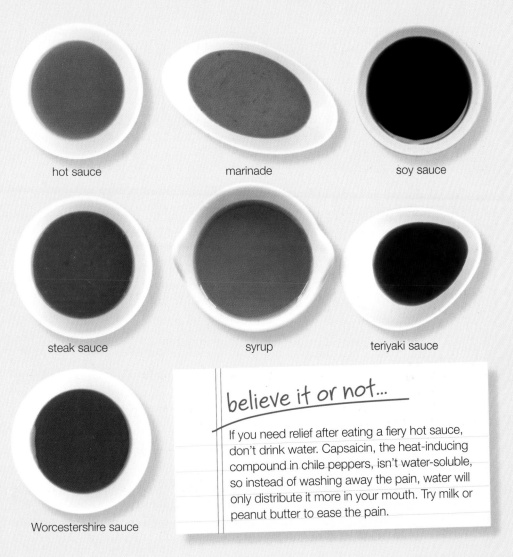

hot sauce

marinade

soy sauce

steak sauce

syrup

teriyaki sauce

Worcestershire sauce

believe it or not...

If you need relief after eating a fiery hot sauce, don't drink water. Capsaicin, the heat-inducing compound in chile peppers, isn't water-soluble, so instead of washing away the pain, water will only distribute it more in your mouth. Try milk or peanut butter to ease the pain.

jams & jellies

Sweet jams, jellies, and preserves are a flavorful addition to an array of meals—from your morning breakfast toast to the classic PB&J.

the healthiest choice

Jams, jellies, and preserves contain no fat and little sodium, and at an average of 40 calories per tablespoon, they can add a boost of flavor to a plain piece of toast. Some may be high in sugar, so if you're closely watching your calories, opt for a low-sugar (25 calories per tablespoon) or no-sugar-added (10 calories per tablespoon) variety to help keep your diet in check.

peanut butter

Crunchy or creamy? On the peanut butter aisle, the choice is no longer this simple. With labels claiming "low-sugar," "low-sodium," and "no trans fats," the options have become more complicated. Follow these simple tips to make the decision easier.

the healthiest choice

On average, 1 tablespoon of full-fat peanut butter has 100 calories and 8 grams of total fat. While that fat count may seem high, the majority of it is good-for-your-heart unsaturated fats. One tablespoon also contains almost 4 grams of quality protein. Be sure to go for the real deal. The reduced-fat spreads offer little calorie savings, and you're losing healthy fats. Plus, the full-fat varieties trump reduced-fat flavor, so choose a brand whose flavor you prefer. Just watch out for trans fats (see the red flag on page 174).

peanut butter, continued

 Watch out for partially hydrogenated oils.

These oils add unhealthy trans fats to a product. To avoid them, you can check the nutrition label to see that the trans fats are listed as zero, but you'll also need to read the ingredient list and make sure "partially hydrogenated oils" aren't included. If they are, then the product contains some trans fats. By law, food companies aren't required to list how many grams of trans fat an item contains if it's less than 0.5 grams per serving, so a product may still contain trace amounts.

fyi other nut butters

There are an array of tasty nut butters available—from cashew and almond to hazelnut and pistachio. Their nutritional properties mimic the nuts they are made from, meaning they are filled with healthy fats and filling protein.

Q&A What is natural peanut butter?

Natural peanut butters are made using peanuts, salt, and maybe sugar. That's it. The only catch is that without the added fat component to prevent separation, there will be a layer of oil sitting on top. You just need to give the peanut butter a good stir before using it, and then store it in the refrigerator.

best crunchy
Jif® Extra Crunchy and Skippy® Super Chunk

We liked both these brands. Jif had a nice crunch and a balanced flavor, while Skippy had an abundance of nuts and a pleasantly salty taste.

best creamy
Skippy® Creamy

The roasted peanuts on the ingredient list are evident in the balanced flavor and aroma. We thought it was a little oily, but it spreads with the least effort to make the perfect peanut butter sandwich.

best natural creamy
Adams® 100% Natural Creamy

Even though you expect a little graininess from natural butters, this brand's consistency smoothed out nicely after a good stir, revealing a mild peanut flavor.

best natural crunchy
Krema® Natural Crunchy

The label claims no added sugar, salt, or hydrogenated oils, and we didn't miss the sweetness or savoriness. We liked the hunks of peanuts, the crunch, and the real peanut flavor.

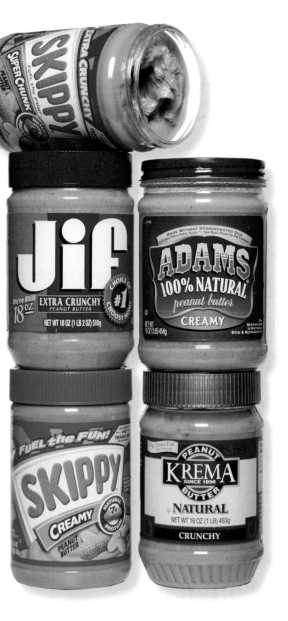

salad dressings

Salads dressings can add loads of flavor to any bowl of healthy greens, but there can be more to that bottle of dressing than you think.

the healthiest dressings

Opting for low-fat and fat-free dressings is really a smart move. By substituting them for full-fat favorites, you can save 100 calories and 14 grams of fat or more per serving. Most brands have a lower-fat alternative, such as a low-fat or fat-free option, that provides a ton of flavor without all the fat and calories. Try a variety of brands to find the one you prefer, and try to choose one that has 40 calories or less and less than 0.5 grams of saturated fat per tablespoon.

Oil and vinegar-based dressings are generally low in calories and high in healthy fats.

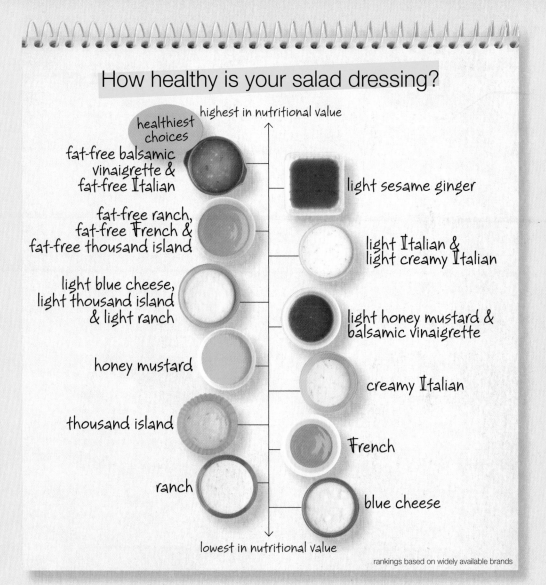

How healthy is your salad dressing?

highest in nutritional value

healthiest choices

fat-free balsamic vinaigrette & fat-free Italian

light sesame ginger

fat-free ranch, fat-free French & fat-free thousand island

light Italian & light creamy Italian

light blue cheese, light thousand island & light ranch

light honey mustard & balsamic vinaigrette

honey mustard

creamy Italian

thousand island

French

ranch

blue cheese

lowest in nutritional value

rankings based on widely available brands

prepared salads

Don't assume that everything with the word "salad" in it is healthy. While some ready-made salads may have certain nutritional benefits, many don't, and it can be hard to tell the difference.

the healthiest prepared salads

Prepared tuna salads, chicken salads, and shrimp salads are often loaded with hidden fats and calories due to the amount of full-fat mayonnaise they contain. For the healthiest choice, opt for salads made with low-fat mayonnaise, and keep the portion size to about the size of a deck of cards.

Ideally, a ½-cup serving of a protein-based salad (like chicken, tuna, or egg salad) will contain less than 200 calories and less than 1 gram of saturated fat per serving, while a vegetable-based prepared salad (like potato) will have less than 100 calories and 0.5 grams of saturated fat per ½ cup. Better yet, instead of those ready-made grocery-store salads, make your own at home so you know exactly what's in it.

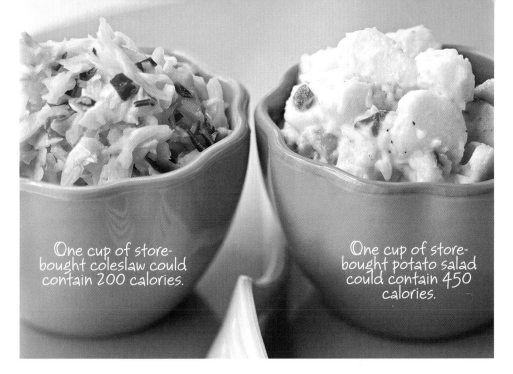

One cup of store-bought coleslaw could contain 200 calories.

One cup of store-bought potato salad could contain 450 calories.

coleslaw and potato salad

The store-bought varieties of these American classics can pack in a lot more than you bargained for. In general, coleslaw beats potato salad in having lower calories and fat. At their base, these salads do provide some nutritional benefits. Cabbage, the main ingredient in coleslaw, is an excellent source of cancer-fighting phytochemicals, and potatoes are an excellent source of potassium.

fyi unhealthy salads

While a lot depends on portion size and the ingredients, an overstuffed tuna salad sandwich can contain as much as 700 calories and 40 grams of fat.

dips

Fruit, vegetable, and bean-based dips flavored with spices instead of salt are the healthiest options out there.

the healthiest dips

Choose prepared dips that have fruit, vegetables, beans, and legumes as their primary ingredients (they'll be listed first in the ingredient list) and are filled out with low-fat dairy, healthy oils (see page 184), and nuts for an additional nutrient boost. For example, salsa is made only of vegetables and is low in both calories and fat. Creamy hummus is another healthy option; it contains healthful fats from olive oil and tahini (sesame seed paste). Always check the nutrition label, since some dips can contain unexpected ingredients that can make them more calorie dense than expected.

pesto

Even though it's made with high-calorie ingredients like nuts, olive oil, and cheese, pesto is a healthful spread. One tablespoon supplies a reasonable 58 calories and 5 grams of good-for-you unsaturated fat.

Tasty premade refrigerated pestos offer basil, Parmesan, garlic, and olive oil flavors in one healthy, handy ingredient.

dips, continued

salsa and guacamole

These Mexican favorites provide a variety of nutritional benefits. Two tablespoons of salsa is skinny on calories and has no fat, while the same amount of guacamole is higher on both counts, but most of the fat is the heart-healthy unsaturated kind. Both are also rich sources of vitamins and minerals; avocados have more vitamin E than any other fruit, while a single tomato offers 40% of the recommended daily allowance of vitamin C. It's easy to find a variety of salsa options on the grocery store shelves, but guacamole may be a bit harder. The tubs of guacamole you'll see in the refrigerated section don't usually contain much actual avocado. The best way to ensure you get the nutritional benefits is to make your own or buy a brand that has avocado listed as its first and primary ingredient. Either way, go easy on fried tortilla chips. Serve baked chips instead.

condiments, dips & oils

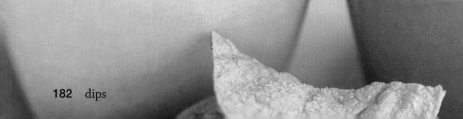

Watch out for the dippers you select.

Don't forget that you won't generally be eating dips unaccompanied. You'll need to consider that you'll be adding crackers, chips, or fresh vegetables to the serving plate. Fresh fruits and vegetable are always the healthiest choice to serve as dippers, but sometimes they just won't cut it. See pages 246 and 248 for more information about how to select healthy crackers and chips.

oils

Oils may be 100% fat, but their heart-healthy properties give them a place in a healthful diet.

the healthiest oils

The fact that oils are 100% fat translates to 120 calories per tablespoon. The fat content is made up of varying proportions of monounsaturated, polyunsaturated, and saturated fats (see below for the exact percentages). An ideal all-purpose oil is low in saturated fats and high in mono- and polyunsaturated fats. Our favorites are olive and canola oils. There is no substitute for the bitter-fruity flavor of olive oil. Canola oil has the least amount of saturated fat of any cooking oil, and its mellow, adaptable flavor makes it perfect for a wide range of uses. Oils labeled simply as "vegetable oils" can be another healthy option, since they're usually made of soybean oil. Check the ingredient list of the vegetable oil you're buying to be sure.

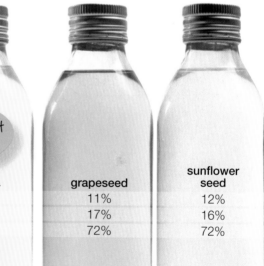

healthiest choice

	canola	grapeseed	sunflower seed
saturated fat	7%	11%	12%
monounsaturated fat	61%	17%	16%
polyunsaturated fats	32%	72%	72%

> ## Oils with high levels of mono- or polyunsaturated fats offer the most health benefits.

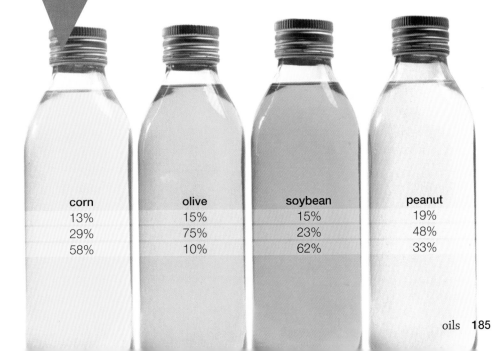

corn	olive	soybean	peanut
13%	15%	15%	19%
29%	75%	23%	48%
58%	10%	62%	33%

oils, continued

specialty oils

These oils can really rev up the flavor of certain dishes. And if used in moderation, you can avoid unnecessary added fat.

truffle-infused oil

This oil rarely contains true truffle (it's usually made with chemical compounds), but it provides a budget-friendly way to impart expensive truffle flavor to dishes.

Per tablespoon: 118 calories, 13.8g fat (2g sat fat)

unfiltered extra-virgin olive oil

This oil may contain small bits of olives, which intensify the flavor. However, those bits can become rancid quickly. It's best to buy this oil in small quantities and use within three to six months.

Per tablespoon: 120 calories, 14g fat (2g sat fat)

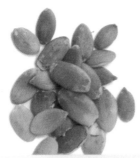

pumpkinseed oil

This expensive oil extracted from Austrian pumpkins has a slightly bitter but pleasing nutty flavor.
Per tablespoon: 120 calories, 14g fat (3g sat fat)

walnut oil

Walnut oil is rich in plant-based omega-3 fatty acids.
Per tablespoon: 120 calories, 13.6g fat (1.2g sat fat)

toasted sesame oil

This bold, roasted seasoning oil is often used to finish Chinese and Japanese dishes.
Per tablespoon: 120 calories, 14g fat (2g sat fat)

canned & boxed foods

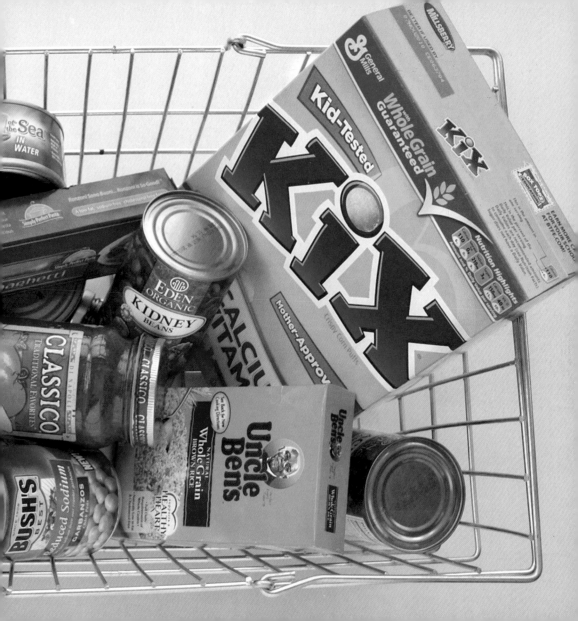

canned &
boxed foods

Why eat canned and boxed foods?

They're quick and convenient, and they can also provide important nutrients, such as:

☑ healthy fats
☑ fiber
☑ protein
☑ vitamins
☑ minerals

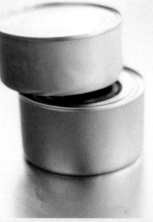

How much should I eat?

For fruits and vegetables (whether canned, fresh, or frozen), the Dietary Guidelines recommend adults eat anywhere from 5 to 13 servings per day depending on age, gender, physical activity, and overall health.

Grains and pastas follow the same guidelines as breads—the amount you need to eat depends on your age, gender, and level of physical activity, but most adults and children need 5 to 8 servings, and at least half of those should be whole grains.

There's not a specific recommendation for meats, poultry, and seafood, just a protein recommendation. While the amount you need depends on your age, gender, and level of physical activity, most adults need about 1 to 1½ servings (the equivalent of 5 to 6½ ounces of cooked protein) per day. For healthy adults, consuming more protein in a day shouldn't be a health concern.

What is a serving?

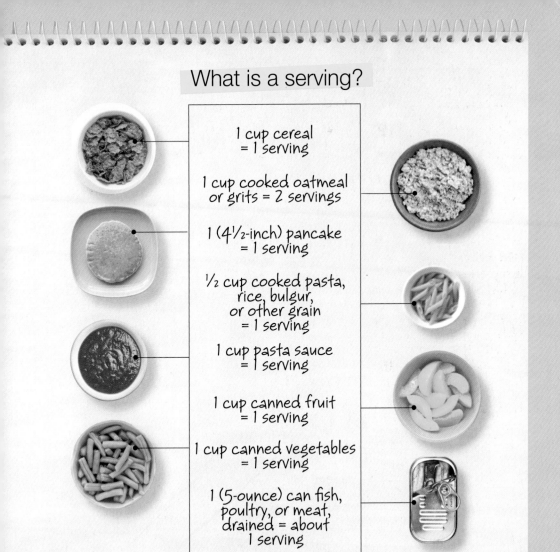

1 cup cereal
= 1 serving

1 cup cooked oatmeal
or grits = 2 servings

1 (4½-inch) pancake
= 1 serving

½ cup cooked pasta,
rice, bulgur,
or other grain
= 1 serving

1 cup pasta sauce
= 1 serving

1 cup canned fruit
= 1 serving

1 cup canned vegetables
= 1 serving

1 (5-ounce) can fish,
poultry, or meat,
drained = about
1 serving

choose the healthiest canned & boxed foods

These aisles provide a bevy of convenient options, and they can be healthy, too, if you know what to look for.

1. Choose whole grains.

When buying pastas, grains, and cereals, select whole grains or those made with whole grains. A whole grain includes the germ, endosperm, and bran, a trio that offers antioxidants, vitamins, and minerals as well as fiber. The USDA recommends that half the grain servings you eat daily should come from whole grains. One way to easily identify items with whole grains is to look for the FDA health claim on the package as well as the stamp created by the Whole Grains Council, a nonprofit group that helps identify whole-grain foods. For more information about identifying whole grains, see page 69.

WHOLE GRAIN
8g or more per serving
WholeGrainsCouncil.org
EAT 48g OR MORE OF WHOLE GRAINS DAILY

2. Look for cereals that are fortified.

While it's best to get all your vitamins and minerals naturally from a variety of foods, some days that's just not possible. Many ready-to-eat cereals are fortified with iron, folate, calcium, vitamin D, or a combination of those that can help you meet your daily needs. However, you should note that some unhealthy cereals use the fact that they're fortified as a health claim on their packaging. Follow our guidelines on page 196 to make sure the cereals you are buying are indeed healthy.

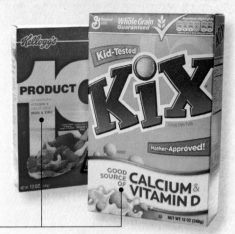

3. Choose "no-salt-added" and "less-sodium" options when available.

More and more food manufacturers are creating no-salt-added or less-sodium products, which are certainly beneficial, since our diets tend to be overly salty. You should know that the term "less-sodium" doesn't necessarily mean the food is low in sodium—it simply means the product contains less sodium than the original. Always check the label: Some products that are lower in sodium may not be listed that way (such as organic products), and some that say they are lower in sodium may not contain the least amount. Always compare labels and find the one with the lowest amount per serving.

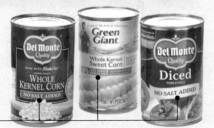

watch out for these red flags

These easy-to-prepare foods can simplify your life in the kitchen, but unfortunately not all of them do the same for your health. Here are the primary things to watch out for in convenience items.

> About 75% of our salt intake comes from processed foods, not from the salt shaker.

Watch out for sodium.

Very little of the sodium we consume arrives in our diet via salt shakers. The majority of sodium—about 75%—comes from processed foods, where it enhances flavor and acts as a stabilizer or a preservative. Boxed and canned foods are some of the high-sodium culprits. Read the labels to find good choices, such as less-sodium or no-salt-added products, and follow our sodium suggestions throughout this chapter.

⚑ Watch out for serving sizes.

Sometimes your idea of a serving might not be the same as what's listed on the package. Manufacturers may list a small serving size that at first glance gives the impression that the calories, saturated fat, and sodium are reasonable. However, if you double or triple the amount to what you consider to be a normal serving, those numbers don't look so pretty.

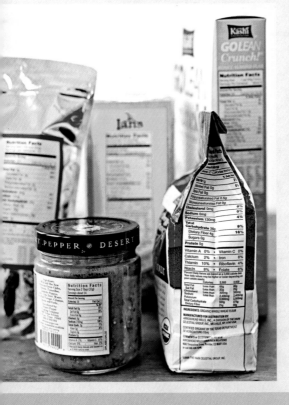

⚑ Watch out for partially hydrogenated oils.

Partially hydrogenated oils can hide in the strangest of places, so you really have to be on the lookout for them. The package may say "trans fat free," but that's not always entirely true. (By law, a product can claim to be trans fat free if it has less than 0.5 grams of trans fat *per serving*.) Check the ingredient list to be sure you don't see "partially hydrogenated oil." If you do, it has trans fats, despite what the label claims.

cereals

The choices on the cereal aisle are astounding. Here's what you need to know to choose wisely.

the healthiest choice

Many cereals on the grocery store shelves are loaded with sugar and contain virtually no fiber or vitamins and minerals—they essentially provide only calories and no nutritional value. But there are some excellent options available. The best choice is a whole-grain variety that's low in sugar and sodium and provides some fiber and iron. As a general recommendation, look for cereals, including granola, that contain 150 calories or less, 9 grams of sugar or less, at least 2 grams of fiber (the more, the better), and 210 milligrams of sodium or less per serving. Also look for fortified cereals when possible—you'll find them fortified with iron, folate, calcium, and vitamin D. They can help you meet your needs when your diet isn't up to par.

Watch out for added sugars.

Some types of cereals are loaded with sugar—certain ones have more than 50% sugar—and have very little fiber. While sugar provides flavor in these cereals, it provides no nutritional benefits.

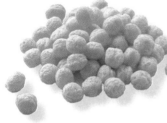

best kids' cereal

 Kix®

Kix has some whole grains (whole-grain corn is the second ingredient on the list, after cornmeal). Plus, it doesn't add extra sugary calories with fruit or yogurt clusters, mini cookies, or candy bits. For a slightly sweetened cereal, this is one you can feel good about feeding your kids (or having some yourself).

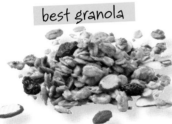

best granola

 Mona's® Original Granola

Seeds and nuts make regular granola a good source of good fats. While low-fat granola sounds like it would be a healthy choice, it has actually had these good fats removed. In Mona's Original Granola, you'll find A-list ingredients—sunflower seeds, wheat germ, almonds, dried fruit, and whole-grain oats—and not a speck of trans fat.

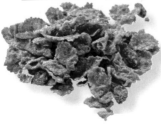

best flake cereal

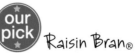 Raisin Bran®

This classic choice sits smartly in the middle between plain flakes and overly accessorized blends. It ups the flavor factor with raisins, even as it keeps it real nutritionally. The first ingredient is whole wheat, so you get all the nutritional benefits of whole grain plus a fiber bonus from the raisins and wheat bran.

oatmeal

Oatmeal has *many* nutritional benefits, from reducing cholesterol levels to helping control weight.

nutritional benefits

Oatmeal is a whole grain that's rich in soluble fiber (specifically beta-glucans), which can improve heart health by reducing LDL cholesterol levels, help with weight control by keeping you feeling fuller longer, and may lower your risk for developing type 2 diabetes by preventing dramatic spikes in blood sugar. It also provides a healthy dose of iron.

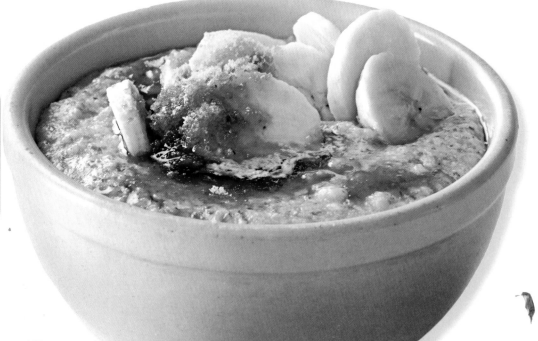

types of oats

Some welcome news is that the basic rolling and cutting process used to make instant and quick varieties does not damage the nutrition. So whether you want quick convenience or a slow-cooked nutty bowl of groats, it's all good.

regular (rolled)

What most of us know as oatmeal is made of whole groats that have been steamed and then flattened by large rollers. They're ready in about 5 minutes.

instant

These are regular rolled oats that are flattened even more, then cooked and dried. (Don't confuse these with sugary pulverized instant oat packets.)

oat groats

Oats as nature intended (they're similar to wheat berries). You'll need about 45 minutes of stovetop simmering before they're tender.

steel-cut (Irish)

These are whole groats that have been halved or cut into three pieces, so they cook faster (about 20 minutes) and the finished dish is chewier.

oatmeal, continued

healthy additions

Amp up the flavor of your bowl with healthy stir-ins. Swirl, sprinkle, or top with any one of these options for less than 100 calories each.

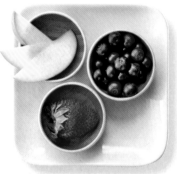

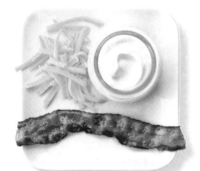

- 2 tablespoons diced apple
- ¼ cup sliced strawberries
- ¼ cup blueberries

- ½ slice of bacon, crumbled
- 1½ tablespoons shredded cheese
- ¼ cup nonfat Greek yogurt

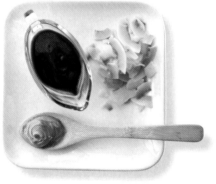

- 1 tablespoon peanut butter
- 1 tablespoon toasted coconut
- 1 tablespoon chocolate syrup

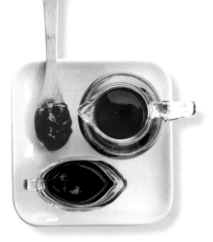

- 1 tablespoon strawberry jam
- 2 teaspoons maple syrup
- 1 teaspoon molasses

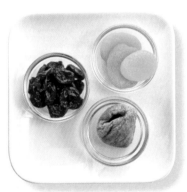

- 1 tablespoon dried cherries
- 1 tablespoon diced and dried apricots
- 1 tablespoon diced and dried figs

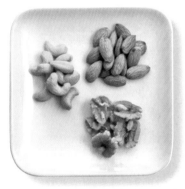

- 1 tablespoon sliced almonds
- 1 tablespoon chopped cashews
- 1 tablespoon chopped walnuts

grits

All grits are not the same—choosing the right kind means you'll get more health benefits.

what to look for

Grits are coarsely ground corn, and depending on how they're milled, they can be another source of whole grains. Grits that are conventionally milled usually lose most of their nutrients during processing when the nutrient-rich bran and germ are removed leaving just the carbohydrate-rich endosperm. However, if you choose a stone-ground variety, the milling process is slower, and more vitamins and minerals are retained. Avoid the instant packs, since they often have added flavorings and salt.

baking mixes

Pancakes, waffles, and biscuits are breakfast favorites, and there are options available to make them healthier.

what to look for

There are a number of healthier all-purpose baking mixes out there that are lower in calories and saturated fat than their traditional counterparts. The primary difference between them is the type of oil that's used. Traditional mixes often use unhealthy partially hydrogenated oils, while the healthier versions use canola oil, which means they're lower in saturated fats and don't contain any trans fats (hence, the "heart healthy" claim on the package). Others will add whole-wheat flour and inulin (see page 83) to the mix to help bump up the fiber content. These small changes make a noticeable and important difference in the nutritional content without drastically affecting the flavor or texture of your baked products. Choose either of these baking mixes (the heart-healthy variety or the one with more fiber), or, if you can find it, a brand that incorporates both.

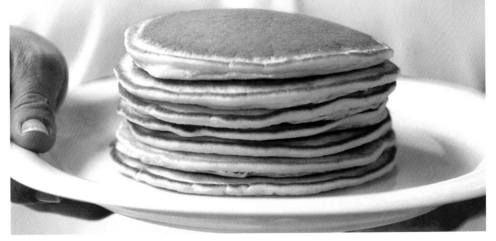

cake & brownie mixes

These convenient mixes usually just require the addition of water, oil, and maybe an egg. But you'll need to read the label closely to know what you're actually getting in that box.

what to look for

Cake and brownie mixes are an easy way to whip up a sweet treat. But remember, since these are treats, you should enjoy them in moderation. When you are selecting a brand, the primary concern is trans fat. Be sure to read the ingredient list closely to make sure "partially hydrogenated oils" aren't included in the mix. There are a number of widely available brands that don't contain any trans fats, so once you narrow down your choices among those, feel free to choose the one with the flavor you prefer.

Watch out for the type of oil that you use.
These may be treats, but it's still important to use a healthful oil that's lower in saturated fat. Go for a neutral-flavored oil, such as canola oil, that won't impart a strong flavor to your baked goods.

breakfast bars

Approach breakfast bars with a wary eye. Some offer lots of nutritional benefits, while others offer anything but. You'll need to study the package to figure out which is which.

what to look for

Breakfast bars are convenient, but not all are healthy. Some are filled with protein and fiber that can keep you full until lunchtime, while others are packed with sugar—you'll get a sugar high that will fade well before noon. You need to read the label to make sure these grab-and-go breakfast options are a good way to start your day. Choose ones with no more than 15 grams of sugar, at least 5 grams of protein, and a minimum of 5 grams of fiber per serving. The fiber will keep you full and help your heart.

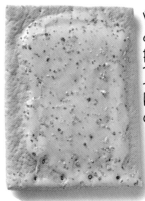

With 19 grams of sugar per pastry, it's best to avoid this familiar refined breakfast choice.

⚑ Watch out for "added nutrients."

While health benefits and claims may decorate the fronts of packages, these added nutrients often hide the fact that some products are just junk food. For example, you might get a reasonable amount of added fiber in toaster pastries, but you still get lots of sugar and partially hydrogenated oil. Follow the guidelines at left to decide which breakfast bars fit the bill.

canned fruits, vegetables & beans

Canned fruits and vegetables are a convenient way to meet your daily needs. While there are some things to look out for, these products certainly have a place in a healthy diet.

canned fruits & vegetables

Fruits and vegetables are low in calories and fat and are important sources of fiber, vitamins, and minerals. While it's often thought that fresh is better than canned, canned fruits and vegetables in fact stack up well nutritionally against fresh. Canned produce is often processed shortly after it's harvested. There is some loss of vitamin C from the heat processing during canning, but the other vitamins, minerals, and fiber are retained. If a fruit or vegetable is said to be high in a particular nutrient, then the form (canned, frozen, or fresh) doesn't alter that. However, sodium can be high in canned products, so opt for "no-salt-added" or "less-sodium" varieties. If one isn't available, it's best to buy produce in fresh or frozen forms.

canned fruits, vegetables
& beans, continued

fyi organic

If you're wondering if you should choose organic when purchasing canned fruits, vegetables, and beans, follow the same guidelines you would when buying fresh produce. Those with thin skins or those that aren't peeled before being eaten are the ones most likely to contain trace levels of pesticides. See page 34 for more details. You should note that many canned organic products tend to be lower in sodium, which is a big plus.

USDA ORGANIC

TOMATOES • POMIDORI CUBETTI • DICED TOMATO

Watch out for canned fruit in heavy and light syrups.

You'll often find fruits canned in "light syrup" or "heavy syrup." These sugar-laden mixtures only add calories and flavor to the fruit. Buy only those canned "in juice" to ensure you're getting just the fruit. If those are not available, pick up a fresh or frozen version.

Watch out for added sugars in vegetables.

In addition to sodium (see page 194), manufacturers often add sugars to their canned vegetables for flavor, but these sugars add more than that—they can pack in unnecessary calories. Vegetables aren't a nutrient-dense food, so the calorie levels shouldn't be sky-high.

canned fruits, vegetables & beans, continued

canned beans

Beans are a great choice, and canned beans offer loads of convenience. They provide a healthy dose of fiber and are a wonderful nonanimal source of protein, which is great for both minimizing saturated fat and for being budget-friendly. But there's no avoiding it: Canned beans contain sodium. Choose "no-salt-added" or "less-sodium" beans to minimize the sodium, and be sure to check the labels as different brands can vary. You can also reduce the sodium by draining the beans and then rinsing them in a colander before using. This simple step reduces the sodium by 40%.

> **Draining and rinsing canned beans reduces the sodium content by 40%.**

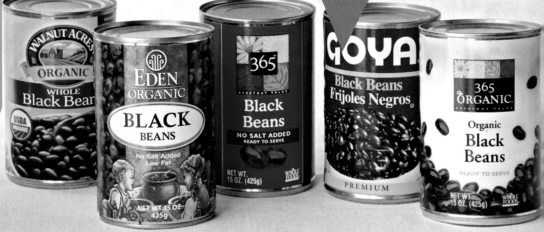

dried beans

Dried beans offer the same fiber and protein as their canned counterparts with the advantage of no added sodium.

nutritional benefits

Beans are rich in fiber and protein and low in saturated fat. And the dried form is a fantastic option when compared to canned because you control how much, if any, sodium you add. They're budget-friendly, too.

pasta sauces

Supermarket shelves are groaning with jarred pasta sauces. While some sauces may appear the same on the outside, the contents inside can be dramatically different nutritionally.

what to look for

Instead of creamy white sauces, choose tomato-based sauces, which are lower in calories and provide valuable nutrients, including potassium; vitamins A, C, and K; and the antioxidant lycopene. But if a white sauce is really what you want, many brands now offer light and reduced-fat versions that can be a healthier substitute. However, for all pasta sauces, you need to be mindful of sodium and choose one that contains less than 700mg of sodium per ½-cup serving.

Watch out for bottled Alfredo sauces.

The jarred creamy, full-fat Alfredo sauces can be *loaded* with calories, saturated fat, and trans fat. Choose a light version and watch your portion size.

Watch out for major variations between brands.

You may need to try a few different sauces before you find one you like as there can be variations among brands nutritionally as well as differences in consistency (from watery to pasty) and flavor (from not enough flavor to overpowering).

canned & boxed foods

our pick Bove's® Basil Pasta Sauce 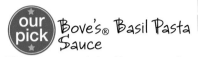 very good

This sauce contains Parmesan cheese that is combined with an herby flavor to give it a pizzeria quality.

our pick Emeril's® All Natural Tomato & Basil Pasta Sauce good

This sauce has a sweetness with a subtle basil taste, but it also has great tomato flavor and a smooth texture.

our pick Rao's® Homemade Tomato Basil Marinara Sauce best

At $9 a jar, this is a pricier choice, but it struck us as very fresh tasting. It's a good choice for a special-occasion dinner in which you want homemade flavor without the time investment.

 our pick Classico® Tomato & Basil Pasta Sauce budget pick

This sauce has a garlicky flavor in a slightly thinner tomato-based sauce. Basil makes only a minor appearance, but you could always add fresh basil at home for a more balanced and fresh flavor.

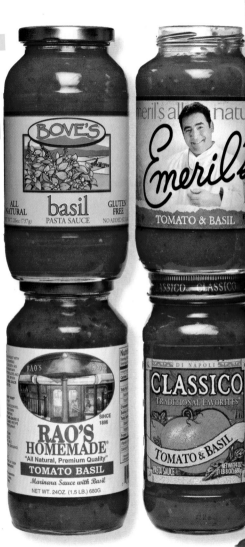
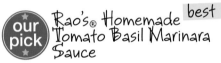

pastas & noodles

Whole-grain pastas are another tasty way to help meet your daily needs for whole grains.

what to look for

The nutritional quality of pasta depends upon the flour that's used, and the best choice is a whole-grain variety—the ones labeled "whole wheat" and that have whole-wheat flour listed first in the ingredient list. Unlike refined pastas, whole-grain noodles don't lose their bran and germ during processing, which is important because the bran and germ carry healthy fats, protein, antioxidants, B vitamins, minerals, and fiber. This mix of nutrients may lower the risks for diabetes, heart disease, and cancer. The USDA recommends at least half of the grains you eat daily should come from whole grains. Filling the quota with whole-grain breads, oatmeal, and cereals are options, but whole-grain pastas offer another tasty way. If you're not ready to go completely whole grain with your pasta, start with a whole-grain pasta blend. The mix of regular pasta with whole grain may be more to your liking. As you get used to it, make the switch to all whole grain.

Whole-grain pasta has more than three times the fiber of refined pasta. That extra fiber keeps you fuller longer.

Pasta is naturally low in fat and sodium. It's the salty, fattening products that we add to it that can make it unhealthy.

pastas & noodles, continued

other types of pasta

You can find a variety of noodles on the pasta aisle—noodles made with buckwheat flour, rice flour, mung bean flour, and potato flour. These bring variety to your diet and can count towards your daily needs for grains, but they are refined grains that don't offer the nutritional benefits of whole grains. Enjoy them, but you'll need to make sure you're meeting your daily needs for whole grains with other foods.

You might also see flavored pastas that include vegetables such as spinach and tomato. These can be an excellent and nutritious substitute for plain pasta.

fyi | egg noodles

Egg noodles are wheat noodles made with egg—the egg adds flavor, color, and texture. Increase the nutritional value by choosing whole-wheat egg noodles.

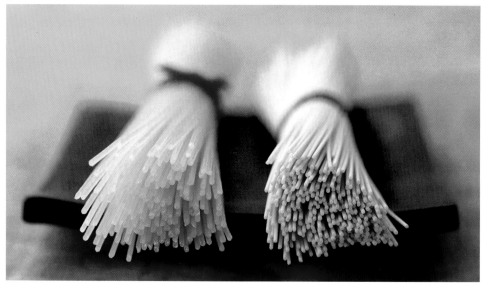

Watch out for boxed pasta mixes.

Those easy boxed mac and cheese mixes and flavored pastas are certainly convenient, but they're often packed with sodium, saturated fat, and calories. If you buy them, choose one of the whole-grain varieties. Be sure to check the ingredient list and choose one that doesn't have "partially hydrogenated oils" listed—you don't need the trans fats those oils provide. Since pasta mixes are also typically dinner favorites, choose one that has the lowest amount of sodium, and watch your portion size. Multiple helpings can add up to *way* too much sodium (and calories and saturated fat).

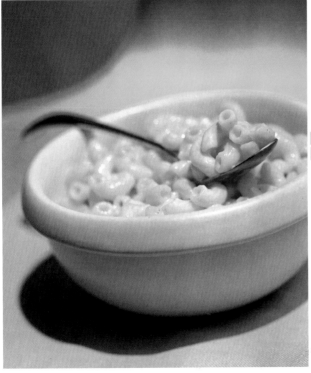

Watch out for instant noodles.

Many of these quick-cooking packages come with flavor packets that are full of sodium. Some of the noodles may be dried by deep frying, so they can be high in fat. It's generally best to avoid them.

dried & boxed grains & lentils

Grains and lentils are packed with slowly digested complex carbohydrates, fiber, and antioxidants. Plus, they're a great way to get in some whole grains.

types of grains

quinoa

This small, round, high-protein grain (pronounced KEEN-wah] is an excellent source of iron—it supplies your entire daily recommendation in 1 cup.

wheat berries

This is a whole-wheat kernel. A ½ cup of cooked berries supplies just 42 calories plus selenium, potassium, folate, and fiber.

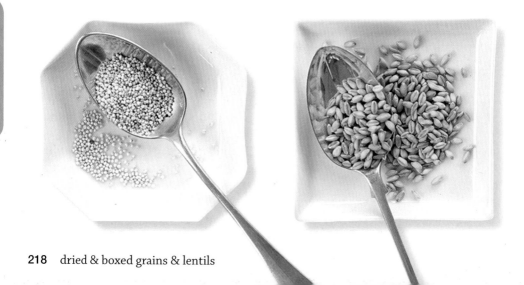

barley

Barley contains a specific kind of fiber called beta-glucans (also found in oats), which may help lower levels of total cholesterol, including artery-clogging LDL cholesterol and blood triglycerides.

buckwheat

A ½-cup serving of cooked buckwheat "groats" contains almost 10% of your daily fiber needs. This is also the only grain that contains the antioxidant rutin, which may help prevent plaque buildup in the arteries.

bulgur

A ½-cup serving of this hearty whole grain contains 4 grams of filling fiber and 30% of your daily needs for manganese, a mineral that supports a healthy metabolism.

millet

This grain offers a host of health benefits. It's an excellent source of manganese, magnesium, and phosphorus.

spelt

Spelt is high in protein—12 grams in ½ cup—and manganese, and it's a good source of fiber, niacin, and magnesium.

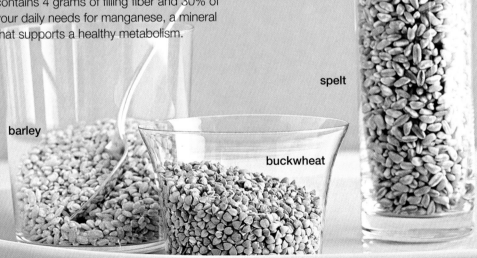

spelt

barley

buckwheat

⚑ Watch out for white rice and flavored mixes.

White rice is simply brown rice that's had the bran covering removed, but you need that bran—it contains fiber (1 cup of brown rice has 3.5 grams of fiber while the same amount of white rice has less than 1 gram). The bran also contains nutrients like magnesium and zinc. White rice has reduced levels of these nutrients but is usually fortified with iron and some B vitamins. And depending on the kind you buy, flavored rice mixes can be very high in sodium. The best bet is to buy plain rice, since it's naturally low in sodium, and then add your own herbs and seasonings. Or look for mixes lower in sodium that contain 300 milligrams or less per ½ cup of cooked rice.

wild rice

This actually isn't a rice at all; instead, it's the seed from a dark brown aquatic grass. It contains insoluble fiber, iron, a host of B vitamins, and vitamin E. It also has fewer calories than brown rice and a healthy dose of folate.

brown rice

This rice provides fiber (mostly insoluble, which aids in digestive health), B vitamins, iron, and vitamin E. A ½-cup serving also provides one-fifth of the daily recommendation for selenium, an antioxidant that helps regulate thyroid function and benefits the immune system.

lentils

Lentils are notably high in protein (a ½-cup serving of cooked lentils contains 8 grams of protein), and they're also a good source of folate, iron, and fiber. Plus, they contribute some B vitamins and zinc.

fyi ## convenience factor

Lentils are one of the oldest cultivated legumes and are sold dried and canned. Unlike dried beans and peas that need to be soaked before cooking and often take more than an hour of simmering to become tender, lentils cook relatively quickly. They're small and flat, so the cooking liquid doesn't have far to penetrate, meaning they can be ready in 40 minutes or less with no need for presoaking. Canned are convenient, but they will be higher in sodium than dried.

Black lentils (also called beluga) sparkle when cooked so that they resemble beluga caviar.

black lentils   green lentils   red lentils   brown lentils

These are the most readily available and most commonly used in the United States.

broths & stocks

Broths and stocks seem simple, but ingredient labels can reveal lots of sodium and frequent use of protein additives and vague flavorings.

what to look for

Purchased broths and stocks can harbor lots of sodium, so read the label and choose one that contains 700 milligrams of sodium or less per cup. Be aware that some broths and stocks meet this criteria but aren't labeled "low-sodium" or "less-sodium." You should also know that the term "less-sodium" doesn't mean it's low in sodium—it means the product contains less sodium than the original.

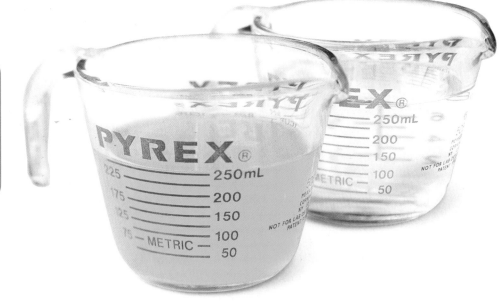

Swanson® Less-Sodium, Fat-Free Chicken Broth

This broth has a pleasant roast chicken flavor and aroma, and at $3 per 32-ounce carton, it won't break the bank either. This is our Test Kitchens' go-to option for recipes.

 Swanson® Certified Organic Vegetable Broth

This broth has a richness and butteriness with a balance of celery, onion, and carrot.

Emeril's® All Natural Chicken Stock

The less-pronounced chicken essence in this stock is balanced with plenty of aromatics. It also has a pleasant saltiness. Though not labeled low-sodium, the sodium count is similar to that of the Swanson low-sodium chicken broth.

 Emeril's® All Natural Organic Vegetable Stock

This broth has a neutral flavor with a slightly sweet aftertaste that makes it a good stock or broth choice.

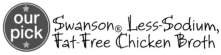

favorite chicken

favorite vegetable

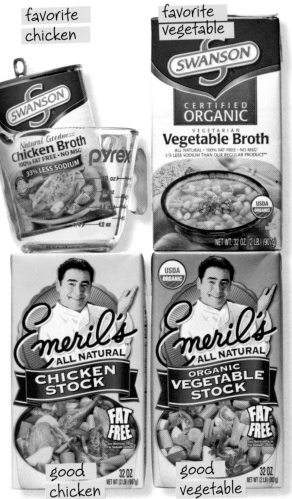

good chicken

good vegetable

canned soups, stews & chili

Canned soups are so easy and convenient: Just open, heat, and eat. But this convenience can come at a nutritional price. Here's what you need to know.

what to look for

Soups, stews, and chili can be easy ways to meet your daily servings of vegetables; however, like most processed foods, the sodium content of these canned products is a concern. To quickly narrow down your picks from the hundreds on the shelves, look for those labeled "lower sodium," "less sodium," or "healthy" and then check the Nutrition Facts label. Be aware, though, that not all healthy soups, stews, and chili—particularly generic or store brands—will have a healthy descriptor, so check those labels closely. They could be beneficial to your health and your budget.

soups

Ideally a 1-cup serving of canned soup should have 250 calories or less, 5 grams of saturated fat or less, at least 2 grams of fiber, and 600 milligrams of sodium or less. Generally, those that are broth-based will be lower in saturated fat and calories.

stews & chili

Stews and chili are heartier than soups, and generally more nutrient dense. Ideally, a 1-cup serving should have 350 calories or less, 8 grams of saturated fat or less, at least 4 grams of fiber, and 800 milligrams of sodium or less.

🚩 Watch out for cream-based soups.

Not all cream-based soups are unhealthy, but you have to read the nutrition label closely to make sure the one you're buying is one of the healthier choices. The problem with these soups can be the saturated fat content, which comes from the cream or dairy product used as the base. Follow our guidelines on page 224 to help you make the healthiest choice.

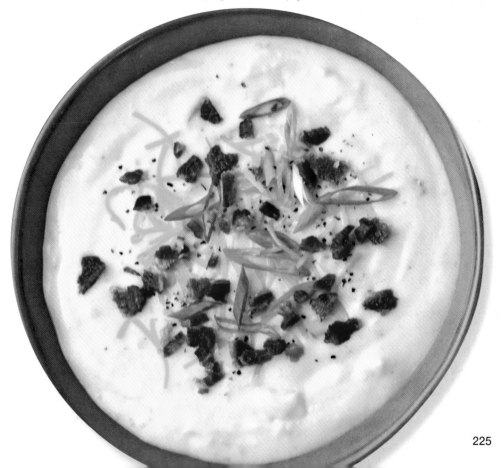

canned seafood, poultry & meats

A variety of seafood, poultry, and meats are available in cans, glass jars, or pouches. It's a convenient and sometimes healthy option. Here's what you need to know.

what to look for

You can find a variety of seafood, poultry, and meats in cans, tins, glass jars, or pouches. They're available year-round and provide a convenient and quick source of high-quality protein. These proteins come packed dry or in liquids, such as water, broth, oil, or oil-based marinades. The best choices are those packed dry or in water or their own cooking juices, which doesn't add unnecessary saturated fat or calories. Read the ingredient list on the label to see if salt or any other ingredients have been added, and avoid those products.

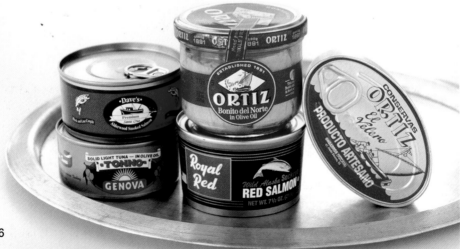

sustainable seafood

If you're concerned about sustainability, look for the blue Certified Sustainable Seafood logo developed by the Marine Stewardship Council. (See page 93 for more details.) You can find it on package labels, in grocery stores and shops that sell seafood, and in restaurants. But this seal isn't on all sustainable products, so do your homework on the sustainable seafood available in your area.

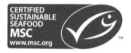

omega-3s

Both canned tuna and canned salmon are sources of omega-3 fatty acids. Tuna varieties differ in the amounts of omega-3s they provide. Albacore, often labeled "white meat tuna," has the most—one 4-ounce serving packed in water delivers 1.1 grams, while you'll get 0.5 gram from the same size serving of albacore packed in oil. Since omega-3s are oils, they don't disperse when the fish is packed in water, and draining the water allows most of these beneficial fatty acids to remain in the fish. But when tuna is packed in oil, the fish's natural oils mix with the packing oils, so when the can is drained, some of the omega-3s go down the drain, too. In canned salmon, there is no significant difference in omega-3 levels among varieties—a 4-ounce serving contains 2.2 grams.

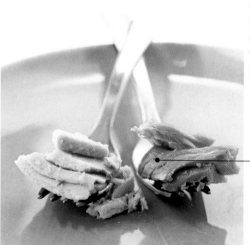

Canned salmon contains soft, edible bones that give it 15 times more calcium than canned tuna.

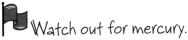 # Watch out for mercury.

All seafood contains trace levels of mercury, but some have higher concentrations that can be harmful to unborn children and young children. As a result, the Food and Drug Administration and the Environmental Protection Agency advise pregnant women, women who may become pregnant, nursing mothers, and young children to avoid some types of fish and shellfish and to only eat seafood with lower levels of mercury. Those with the highest levels of mercury include shark, swordfish, king mackerel, and tilefish. Salmon and canned light tuna are two fish that are low in mercury, but for at-risk populations, it's best to only eat up to 12 ounces a week of seafood lower in mercury. Albacore "white" tuna has more mercury than canned light tuna, so it's best to eat no more than 6 ounces per week.

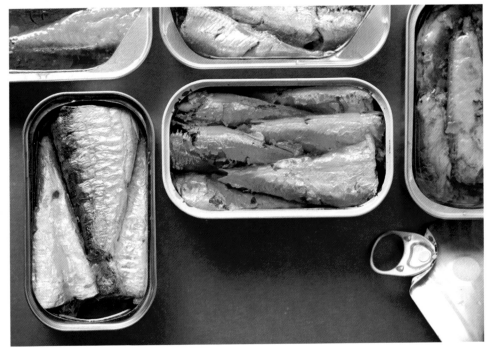

canned poultry

Use the same guidelines you would when making healthy choices about fresh or frozen poultry—for the leanest cut, buy the white meat. Chicken breast packed in water is your best bet, but you'll still need to watch out for sodium. Be sure to check the label and choose the brand that contains the lowest amount.

⚑ Watch out for "meat products."

These canned precooked meats are a combination of various cuts of meats—usually the less healthy cuts that are higher in saturated fat and calories. They also generally have added salt, sugar, and water. The problem with these products is that you really can't be sure what you're getting, so calories and fat can vary widely. Plus, these products are usually high in sodium—even the "lite" or "less-sodium" versions can contain around 600 milligrams of sodium per ¼-cup serving. It's best just to avoid them.

snacks & desserts

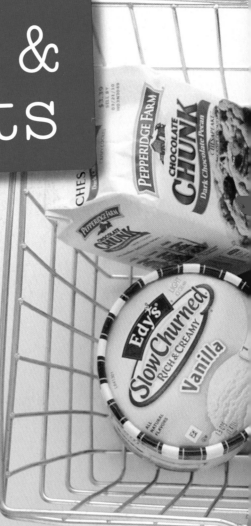

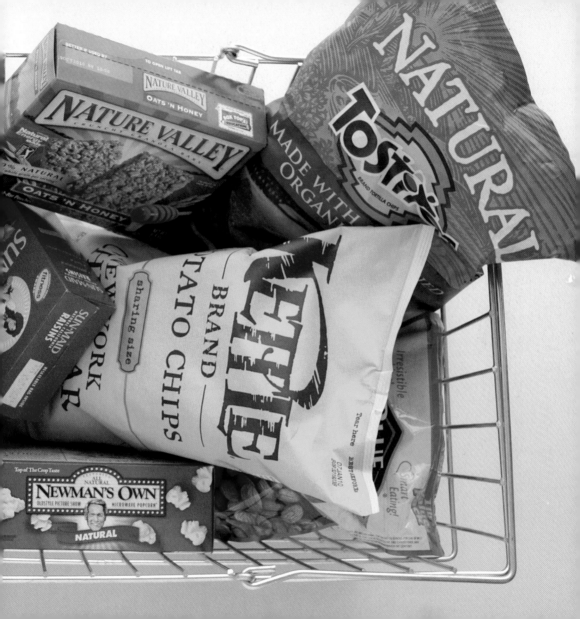

snacks & desserts

Why eat snacks and desserts?

The healthiest snacks can:

- ☑ fill nutritional gaps in your day
- ☑ keep you satisfied between meals
- ☑ provide vitamins, minerals, and antioxidants
- ☑ supply healthy fats
- ☑ help with appetite and weight control

Desserts can:

- ☑ satisfy your all-important sweet tooth

How much should I eat?

The USDA's guidelines for this category of foods vary. For dairy-based snacks and desserts, such as ice cream, frozen yogurt, and puddings, the guidelines of 3 servings of milk or other dairy products per day apply (see page 132). For dried fruits, the guidelines of 5 to 13 daily servings of fruits and vegetables apply (see page 30).

Most other snacks and desserts fall into the discretionary calories category. Each person has a daily allowance of these calories based on their age, gender, and level of physical activity. Most discretionary calorie allowances are very small—between 100 and 300 calories—especially for those who are not physically active. Go to MyPyramid.gov to determine your specific needs.

What is a serving?

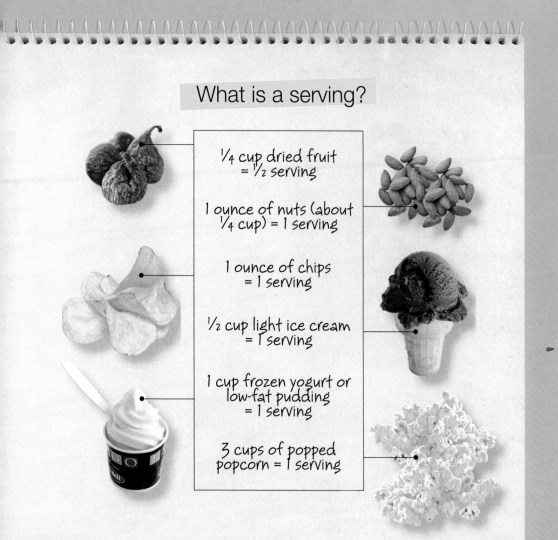

¼ cup dried fruit = ½ serving

1 ounce of nuts (about ¼ cup) = 1 serving

1 ounce of chips = 1 serving

½ cup light ice cream = 1 serving

1 cup frozen yogurt or low-fat pudding = 1 serving

3 cups of popped popcorn = 1 serving

choose the healthiest snacks & desserts

Snacking can help boost your energy levels when you're in an afternoon slump, while desserts are simply a sweet part of life. But when it comes to healthy eating, every bite counts.

1. Choose snacks that contain high-quality protein, complex carbohydrates, and fiber.

When an afternoon energy slump hits, it can be easy to run by the vending machine to quickly grab something. However, many of these choices only offer calories and don't have much nutritional value—plus, some sweet or starchy high-calorie snacks can be the calorie equivalent of a small meal. Instead, choose foods that provide a blend of complex carbohydrates (such as whole grains), high-quality lean protein, and fiber. Complex carbohydrates provide readily available fuel for your body; protein increases the brain's dopamine levels, which boosts alertness; and foods high in fiber are more slowly digested, which will help you stay full longer. Healthful choices like a handful of dried fruit and nuts, a slice of bread with peanut butter, and whole-grain crackers with cheese provide this mix.

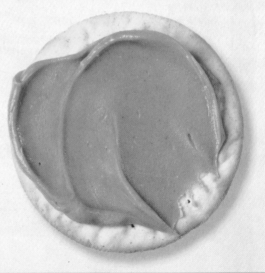

2. Keep portions under control.

Research has shown that people will eat more if a larger portion is offered to them. This can be particularly dangerous with calorie-dense desserts and snack foods that you can grab by the handful. An occasional high-calorie indulgence won't wreck your diet, but regular snackers should pay close attention to the size of the portions they're eating. If portion control is something you struggle with, consider looking for portion-controlled packages, or buy a regular-sized package and portion it into zip-top bags. Your snacking habits should follow the same plan you have for the rest of your diet—everything in moderation.

3. Enjoy your indulgences.

There's a place in every diet for treats, and a healthy approach to eating includes permission to satisfy your cravings for chocolate and ice cream from time to time. Don't feel guilty about indulging—just do so in moderation and enjoy every last bite.

watch out for these red flags

Prepackaged snacks and desserts often come with packaging claims that make healthy choices more complicated. Follow these guidelines to make some sense of the snack aisle.

🚩 Watch out for snacks with "low-fat" or "light" claims.

If a snack or dessert is marked as "low-fat," "reduced-fat," or "light," it doesn't necessarily mean it's low-calorie. That low-fat claim on the package can sometimes give a false sense of security that these foods are somehow safer to eat, which can lead to overeating. Regardless of the fat content, these foods still contain calories, so it's important to treat low-fat foods like any others, and enjoy them in moderation.

🚩 Watch out for sodium.

Prepackaged convenience foods, particularly snacks like chips and crackers, can be very high in sodium per serving. Always read the label and opt for unsalted versions whenever possible.

Watch out for trans fats.

Processed foods can be some of the worst trans fat offenders. These unhealthy fats, which are linked to heart and arterial disease, keep foods fresher longer, which is ideal for foods like cookies and snack cakes. However, even if a package says "trans fat free" or a Nutrition Facts label lists 0 grams of trans fats, that might not always be the case. (See page 195 for more information about trans fats.) Instead, look to the ingredient list and avoid foods that include "partially hydrogenated oils."

Watch out for added sugars.

Added sugars are those that aren't found naturally in foods but are added during processing. They can be from a natural source, such as honey, or from a highly processed source, such as high-fructose corn syrup. While added sugars have a place in our diet, the amount, regardless of type, should be limited because they add empty calories. However, distinguishing added sugar from natural sugar can be confusing, since the nutrition label combines the two and only lists "sugars." Instead, look to the ingredient list. If you see any of the following, then the food contains added sugar: brown sugar, corn sweetener, corn syrup, dextrose, fructose, fruit juice concentrates, glucose, high-fructose corn syrup, honey, invert sugar, lactose, maltose, malt syrup, molasses, raw sugar, sucrose, and sugar syrup.

Nutrition Facts

Serving Size 8 crackers (28g)

Amount Per Serving

		% Daily Value*
Calories 120	Calories From Fat 30	
Total Fat 3.5g		5%
Saturated Fat 1g		5%
Trans Fat 0g		
Polyunsaturated Fat 1.5g		
Monounsaturated Fat 0.5g		
Cholesterol 0mg		0%
Sodium 140mg		6%
Total Carbohy		
Dietary Fiber L		
Sugars 7g		
Protein 2g		
Vitamin A 0%		
Calcium 10%		

This number doesn't tell the whole story. You need to check the ingredient list to be sure a product is trans fat free.

237

granola bars & energy bars

These handy snacks are easy to pick up and go. Just be sure to read the label, since some bars can pack as many calories as a meal.

what to look for

It seems like there are infinite varieties of granola bars and energy bars available, and some have a lot going for them nutritionally: wholesome, whole-grain ingredients; an ingredient list filled with words you recognize and can pronounce; and an outstanding Nutrition Facts label.

However, some aren't so stellar. Watch out for sweet additions, such as chocolate or yogurt coverings, that increase the fat and calories. As a general recommendation, look for bars that have fewer than 200 calories, less than 6 grams of total fat, about 25 to 30 grams of carbohydrates, and 5 to 10 grams of protein.

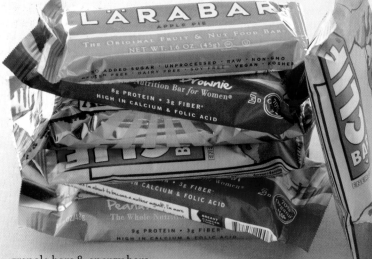

snacks & desserts

nuts

It's OK to go a bit nuts. Nuts are filled with heart-healthy unsaturated fats and a variety of beneficial nutrients.

> An ounce of nuts, the smallest amount that studies show is beneficial, fits neatly into most shot glasses.

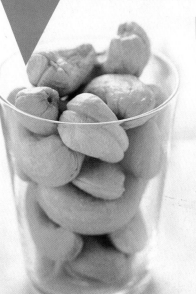

nutritional benefits

Snacking on nuts is a smart choice. They may be mostly fat, but it's primarily the heart-healthy mono- and polyunsaturated kind that can help lower cholesterol. They also contain a variety of other beneficial nutrients, including protein, vitamin E, folate, and magnesium, plus a small amount of fiber and iron. This mix of nutrients also helps keep you full longer, but portion control is key, since the calories in nuts can add up quickly. Aim to eat 1 to 1½ ounces per day—or roughly ¼ to ⅓ cup—enough to cover the palm of your hand.

nuts, continued

types of nuts

Each nut offers its own mix of nutrients. To make sure you're benefitting from all of the nutrients, eat a variety instead of singling out one particular nut to snack on.

Cashews and almonds are good sources of vitamin E, carrying about four to five times more of this antioxidant than other nuts.

Walnuts have the highest amount of omega-3s of any nut.

Pecans have the highest antioxidant capacity of all nuts. They may decrease the risk of cancer, coronary heart disease, and Alzheimer's.

Peanuts have more protein than any other legume or nut, packing in 8 grams in just one (1-ounce) serving.

Pistachios offer more than 30 different vitamins, minerals, and phytonutrients.

Watch out for salt and heavily sugared nuts.

Be mindful when snacking on salted nuts. A 1-ounce serving (about ¼ cup) of salted mixed nuts can contain almost 200 milligrams of sodium. So it's best to forgo that extra salt and opt for the plain roasted varieties. For everyday snacking, don't reduce the nutritional value of nuts by opting for the sugar-coated varieties. Just one serving (about 30 nuts) of some heavily sugared or chocolate-covered nuts can contain 15 grams of sugar per ounce. A healthier choice would be an unsalted variety that contains just 1 gram of sugar.

dried fruits

Dried fruits are a healthful, portable snack, and they have many of the same nutritional benefits as their juicy, fresh counterparts.

nutritional benefits

Dried fruits are a sweet way to help you meet your daily recommendations for fruit (see page 30). A ¼-cup serving—a small handful—counts as one of the two to four servings you need each day.

Watch out for portions.

While dried fruits are an easy snack to grab, you can grab too much. Without the juice, these calories are concentrated, so you should enjoy them in moderation.

snacks & desserts

Adding ¼ cup of dried fruit (like raisins, cranberries, or figs) to your diet counts as one serving of fruit.

trail mix

With the blend of salty and sweet, trail mixes can be the perfect antidote when you're hungry.

nutritional benefits

With the combination of nuts and dried fruits, trail mix is a nutritious sweet-and-salty snack food, but one where portion control is key. A ¼-cup serving contains 194 calories, 3.4 grams of protein, and 9.4 grams of total fat, but more than 80% of that fat is the heart-healthy mono- and polyunsaturated kind. This nutrient mix provides you fuel with staying power.

Watch out for some not-so-healthy additions.

Sweet additions such as chocolate or yogurt clusters increase the calories and fat and give you a lot of extra sugars, so check the label closely when making your selection.

popcorn

Popcorn can be the best or the worst of snacks. It all depends on those buttery and sugary additions.

what to look for

Air-popped popcorn, which has less than half a gram of saturated fat in 3½ satisfying cups, is the healthiest choice out there. Plus, you enjoy a whole-grain serving that's rich in fiber. The 94% fat-free microwave popcorns are nearly as good. However, avoid full-fat microwave popcorn; it contains 4.5 grams of saturated fat and trans fats combined, which can be a significant chunk of your daily limit.

believe it or not...

It's not uncommon for some movie theaters to drench a 7-cup "small" serving with a "buttery topping" that adds 29 grams of saturated fat—almost as much as a behemoth fast-food burger.

Six cups of popcorn—the amount in one single-serving bag—counts as two of the three daily recommended servings of whole grains and provides 5 grams of fiber.

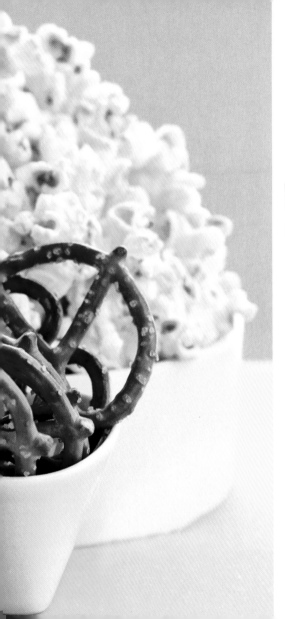

pretzels

Before you open your next bag of pretzels, read the label to find out exactly what's in one serving.

what to look for

For the healthiest choice, choose pretzels that are baked, not fried, and avoid ones that are flavored. Garlic and honey mustard pretzels, for example, have added calories, fat, and sodium. Cheddar pretzels can have up to 6 grams of fat in a single serving, compared to 0 grams of fat in a serving of regular pretzels. A snack-size bag of classic-flavored tiny twist pretzels (about 20 pretzels) contains 110 calories, but just be sure you stick to one serving.

🚩 Watch out for excess salt. With pretzels, which are usually sprinkled with salt, sodium is always a concern. Be mindful of this when selecting a brand and choose one that contains the least amount of sodium per serving—some can contain more then 600 milligrams (more than one-fourth of the daily recommendation) in a 1-ounce serving (about 20 small pretzels).

crackers

Crisp crackers can be the perfect contrast to cheese, peanut butter, and dips. And if you choose a whole-grain variety, they can be a healthy snack, too.

what to look for

Whole-grain crackers are the best choices out there, since whole grains contain complex carbohydrates and fiber, which won't raise blood sugar levels the way refined grains will. However, finding them might be easier said that done amid the blur of claims like "multigrain," "hearty wheat," and "made with whole grains" that you're likely to see on the grocery store aisles. Look to the ingredient list to see that "whole-wheat flour," "whole grain," "whole oats," "whole corn," or "whole rye" (instead of "enriched") is included and listed first or at least very close to the beginning of the list. You can also look for the Whole Grains Stamp developed by the Whole Grains Council to help you easily identify whole-grain products. The stamp doesn't appear on every product that contains whole grains, though. (See page 69.)

100%
WHOLE GRAIN
16g or more per serving
WholeGrainsCouncil.org
EAT 48g OR MORE OF

🚩 Watch out for "wheat."

Just because the package says "wheat" doesn't mean the crackers inside are made with whole-wheat flour. Many wheat crackers are made primarily from enriched (refined) wheat flour, which isn't a whole grain, and they may contain only a little, if any, whole-wheat flour. Some crackers that are labeled as mulitgrain actually only contain about a teaspoon of whole-grain flour in 10 crackers. That's not much.

fyi sweet crackers

Most sweet crackers, like graham and animal crackers, are made with enriched wheat flour or other refined flours. They're fine for an occasional treat, but they don't provide much nutritionally except calories and sugar.

fyi rye crackers

Rye crackers are another healthy choice. They're low in fat, and like oats, rye lowers cholesterol and evens out blood sugar levels for diabetics. Look for crackers made with a mix of rye and whole-wheat flours.

chips

Salty, crunchy chips are easy to eat by the handfuls, but those calories can quickly add up.

what to look for

The downfall of chips is their salty crunchiness that makes it hard to stop eating them once you start. Baked and light varieties are the healthier options, since they offer a calorie savings, and you can also find whole-grain varieties. However, a serving of regular chips won't sabotage a healthy diet. A 1-ounce serving of regular plain potato chips, which is equal to 14 to 28 chips depending on the chip, contains around 150 calories, 1 gram of saturated fat, and 180 milligrams of sodium (and most chips are trans fat free, since they're fried in vegetable oils). But when you multiply that by several handfuls, it can add up to an unhealthy and calorie-laden snack. Regardless of the type you choose, portion control is vital. So pull out a serving and enjoy the crunch.

fyi   corn chips

When you're tired of popcorn as your go-to whole-grain snack, Fritos® Scoops!® are a good alternative: They fit the crunchy, salty snack bill, plus their first ingredient is whole corn. Not bad for a chip.

Q&A Are vegetable chips healthier than other chips?

Most vegetable chips are made from root vegetables, such as sweet potato, taro, parsnip, and yuca, that are fried crisp just like potato chips. However, veggie chips have a slight nutritional advantage over regular potato chips—they usually contain less saturated fat and more fiber. And although they often cost more than potato chips, veggie chips offer real savings in terms of sodium: Most contain one-third of the sodium that usually flavors chips of the spud variety.

chips, continued

snacks & desserts

fyi | bagel chips vs. pita chips

Both bagel chips and pita chips are made from bread and have the same amount of calories and protein per ounce; however, you'll need to look closely at the nutrition label. Some varieties of each can contain a lot of sodium—more than 300 milligrams per 1-ounce serving. Look for whole-wheat versions of both to gain a whole-grain serving and a dose of fiber with your snack.

believe it or not...

Regular fried or kettle-style potato chips have about 10 grams of fat (mostly unsaturated) and 150 calories per ounce— about the size of a single-serving bag. Baked potato chips, made from dried potatoes, binders, and such, have 8 or so fewer grams of total fat than regular but have only 30 or 40 fewer calories.

chocolate

Mounting evidence shows certain forms of chocolate may be good for your health. The key is in the cocoa content.

what to look for

When the right kind is eaten in moderation, chocolate may help reduce high blood pressure, reduce LDL (the "bad cholesterol"), or even provide potential cancer-fighting benefits. It makes sense. Chocolate and cocoa come from a plant—the cacao (pronounced ca-COW)—and contain plant compounds that researchers credit with these health benefits. However, researchers don't attribute these effects to milk chocolate bars or chocolate-coated candies but specifically to dark chocolate and minimally processed cocoa powder—the more cocoa in the chocolate, the more antioxidants it contains. You'll want to avoid highly alkalized, or Dutch processed, as this can significantly reduce the beneficial compounds found in chocolate. Choose dark chocolate with a cocoa content of 70% or more, and limit your portion to about 1.5 ounces. That ensures you'll reap the health benefits without adding too many calories. See page 277 for more information about cocoa.

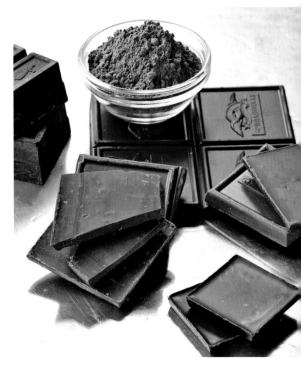

cookies, brownies & snack cakes

Cookies, brownies, and snack cakes are often one of the prime places trans fats are found in the grocery store.

what to look for

Like most desserts, packaged cookies, brownies, and snack cakes can be high in saturated fat, sugars, and calories per serving, so moderation is key. If you eat these products regularly, watch out for those loaded with sugar, and choose those that contain 10 grams or less per serving and preferably as little saturated fat as possible—no more than 1 gram per serving.

snacks & desserts

fyi | chocolate chip vs. oatmeal raisin

If you're deciding between chocolate chip cookies or oatmeal-raisin cookies, opt for the oatmeal. Typical store-brand chocolate chip cookies have 170 calories and 9 grams of fat (3.5 grams saturated fat) in just two cookies compared to 130 calories and 6 grams of fat (2 grams saturated fat) found in the same amount of oatmeal-raisin cookies. Both, however, are high in sugar.

Watch out for trans fats.

Individually wrapped and premade cookies, brownies, and snack cakes can be a jackpot for trans fats—one serving of some of these snacks can contain more than the daily maximum amount of trans fats that the American Heart Association considers safe. The same goes for the treats found in the grocery store bakery. For both, you should make sure the ingredient list doesn't include partially hydrogenated oils. Organic products and those made with all-natural ingredients are usually the best bets. Better yet, make your own from scratch.

frozen yogurt, sorbet & sherbet

These cool treats can be smart choices—especially when chosen in place of ice cream.

what to look for

Frozen yogurt, sorbet, and sherbet are all great choices when eaten in place of full-fat ice cream—we're talking a savings of more than 100 calories and more than 8 grams of saturated fat per ½-cup serving. Sorbets are naturally fat free and generally contain around 120 calories per ½ cup, while a ½ cup of sherbet contains 160 calories. Frozen yogurts are a bit higher—around 200 calories per ½ cup—since the primary ingredient is milk. However, sorbets and sherbets lack the calcium and protein found in frozen yogurt. All are great choices when you're in the mood for something cold and sweet.

A ½-cup portion of nonfat frozen yogurt, made from dairy, provide 4 grams of satiating protein and 15% of your daily calcium requirement.

What's the difference between sorbet and sherbet?

Sorbet is a combination of fruit, juice, and water, making it naturally fat free. Since it contains no dairy, sorbet is ideal for the lactose intolerant. Sherbet is made with the same ingredients as sorbet, but it also contains milk, egg whites, or gelatin.

ice cream

There's nothing like a bowl of ice cream for dessert, and it's not all bad for you either. While many brands are full of fat and sugar, there are plenty of lighter options for you to choose from.

what to look for

Despite the variety of ice cream labels you'll find in the freezer section, buying ice cream doesn't have to be complicated. There are many excellent "light," "fat-free," and "no-sugar-added" ice creams and, cup for cup, each is significantly better for you than full-fat varieties. So when choosing among those healthier versions, you can really let your taste buds be your guide (and you can also use the chart on page 257 to help you). But you should still check the Nutrition Facts labels when you're in the grocery store to be sure the "light" ice cream you're buying really is as light as you think it is.

snacks & desserts

take your pick

We compared ½-cup servings of a variety of vanilla ice creams with varying fat levels. You can see the difference for yourself.

	Regular, full fat	Light	Fat free	No sugar added
Calories	270	110	90	80
Fat	18g	3.5g	0g	4g
Sat fat	11g	2g	0g	2.5g
Sugar	21g	16g	12g	4g
Calcium	15%	10%	10%	6%

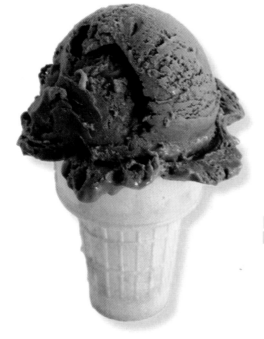

Watch out for sugar alcohols.
Some ice creams, often labeled sugar free or low carb (and sometimes found in no-sugar-added ice creams), contain sugar alcohols, which are used as sweeteners. You'll see them in the ingredient list as mannitol, sorbitol, xylitol, isomalt, maltitol, and hydrogenated starch hydrolysates. As a sugar substitute, they provide fewer calories (about half to one-third less) than regular sugar. However, there are some negatives that you need to be aware of. The most common side effects are bloating and stomach upset when eaten in large amounts. These potential side effects are another reason to watch your portion size.

ice cream, continued

 ## Breyers® Smooth & Dreamy Light Ice Cream

This light ice cream has a creamy texture and a variety of flavors that, at 110 to 140 calories per ½ cup, make eating healthier a whole lot easier.

 ## Edy's® Slow-Churned Light Ice Cream

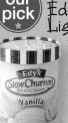

This is our other go-to light ice cream for a flavor and texture that can't be beat.

One ½-cup serving of ice cream has about 10% of the recommended daily amount of calcium.

pudding

Pudding makes a great snack when you're craving something sweet. Pudding packs are easy to grab and go, and most name brands have plenty of healthy options for you to choose from.

what to look for

Pudding labels can be a bit confusing. With healthier "sugar-free" and "fat-free" options and others that promote a 100-calorie serving size, it may not always be easy to decide which is best for you. And really, any of the above are fine choices, since all are portion controlled, have 100 calories or less, and contain minimal fat. For sugar content, the sugar-free variety trumps the others for having 0 grams of sugar in a 60-calorie package (compared to the 17 grams found in the fat-free versions). But for those monitoring their saturated fat content, the sugar-free cups contain 1 gram per serving.

fyi gelatin

When it comes to flavored gelatin snacks, sugar free is the way to go. These little packs have hardly any calories at all—just 10 per cup—and no sugar, while regular gelatin snacks have 70 calories and 17 grams of sugar per cup.

cakes, pies & piecrusts

These convenient desserts are a prime place for trans fats to hide, so pay close attention when purchasing them.

what to look for

The aisle containing premade cakes, pies, and piecrusts is another section that can be a hub for trans fats. These sweet treats are often very high in harmful trans fats. Read the ingredient list, and if you see "partially hydrogenated oil" listed, don't buy it. These treats are high in calories and saturated fat, too, but that's true of many desserts. So find one that's trans fat free and enjoy. Just be sure to practice portion control and make these once-in-a-while indulgences instead of a regular part of your day.

Read the ingredient list. This pie could contain a hefty amount of trans fats.

believe it or not...

Some of the individually wrapped one-serving pies found in the grocery store are *packed* with trans fats—as in, four days' worth. Avoid them.

drinks

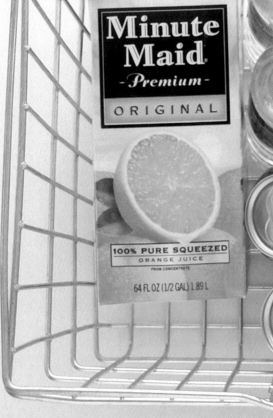

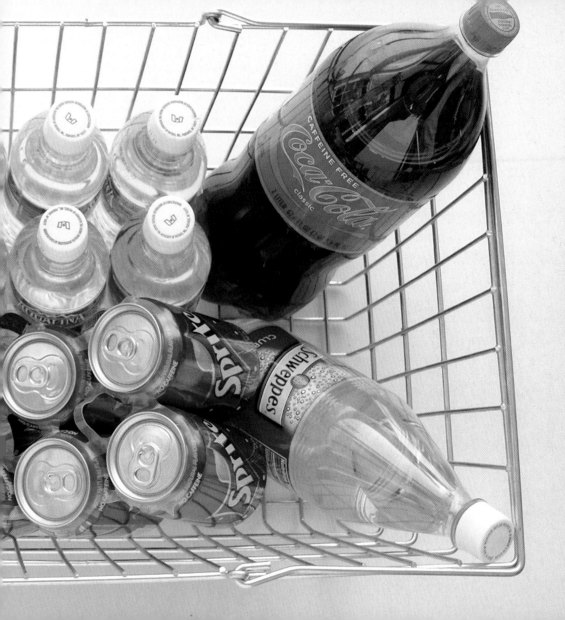

drinks

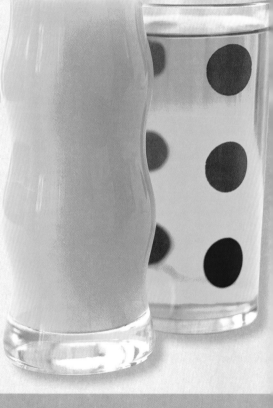

Why drink beverages?

The healthiest drinks:

- ☑ provide hydration
- ☑ supply vitamins, minerals, and antioxidants

How much should I drink?

Optimal hydration depends on your body size, activity level, sweat rate, and climate. Because of that, the Institute of Medicine recommends an Adequate Intake (AI) rather than a specific daily amount. An adequate intake for most women is 2.7 liters or 91 ounces of fluid each day. A man's AI is 3.7 liters or 125 ounces of fluid daily. If you're an avid exerciser or live in a hot climate, you may need more. Most nonalcoholic beverages and even certain foods can help you meet your hydration needs. The serving sizes on page 265 are meant to be a guide for proper portion sizes, since caloric beverages, such as juices and alcohol, should be consumed in moderation. See page 138 for information about milk.

drinks

What is a serving?

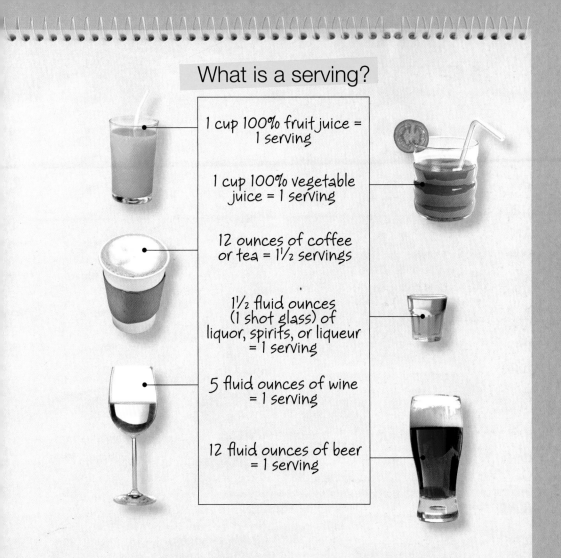

1 cup 100% fruit juice = 1 serving

1 cup 100% vegetable juice = 1 serving

12 ounces of coffee or tea = 1½ servings

1½ fluid ounces (1 shot glass) of liquor, spirits, or liqueur = 1 serving

5 fluid ounces of wine = 1 serving

12 fluid ounces of beer = 1 serving

choose the <mark>healthiest</mark> drinks

Beverages not only help keep you hydrated, but they can also provide valuable nutrients. Here are some things to keep in mind.

1. The less processed the juice, the better.

Pure fruit and vegetable juices have many of the vitamins and minerals of whole fruit, but many "juice drinks," which may look like real juice, can have loads of added sugar and calories and may only contain a tiny bit of juice. In order to get the full nutritional benefits, go for the real deal and choose 100% pure juice.

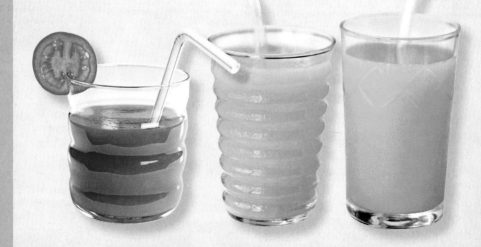

drinks

2. Drink water.

Water isn't the only option for meeting your hydration needs, but it is one of the best, since it's easily accessible, calorie free, and the ultimate hydrator. To make it more flavorful, add a splash of pure fruit juice.

3. Enjoy alcoholic beverages in moderation.

While alcohol does have certain health benefits, those only apply when it's consumed in moderation. An excess amount can undo any benefit alcohol may have provided. A moderate amount of alcohol (wine, beer, liquor, spirits, and liqueur) for women is no more than one serving daily. For men, the limit is two. See page 265 for serving-size guidelines.

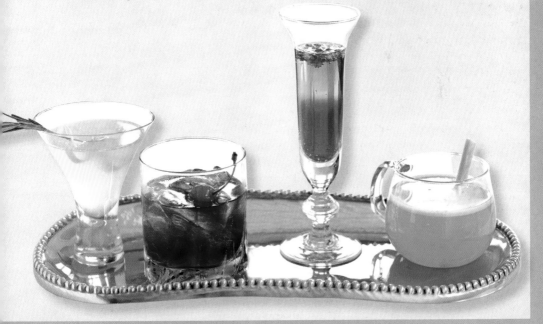

watch out for these red flags

Some beverages don't provide any nutritional benefits whatsoever and can be detrimental to your diet. Here's what you need to avoid.

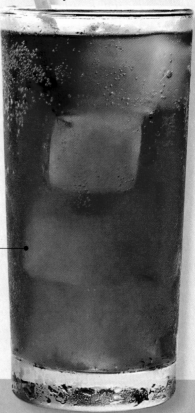

Watch out for sodas.
Regular sodas don't have any redeeming qualities. They're loaded with calories and added sugar, and, when consumed unchecked, can add hundreds of extra calories to your diet that, unlike milk or 100% juice, provide no nutritional benefits.

Regular sodas contain plenty of unnecessary calories that provide no nutritional benefits.

drinks

Watch out for added sugars.

Many juices, sodas, sports drinks, cans of concentrate, and powdered drink mixes contain added sugars that provide flavor but also have lots of unnecessary empty calories. While added sugars have a place in our diet, they still need to be limited. See page 237 for more information about added sugars.

Watch out for portion sizes.

Drinks are often supersized. Whether you're drinking an individually bottled juice or soda or a fountain drink from a restaurant, you're likely consuming well more than one serving. The average individual bottle of juice is 16 ounces or 2 servings, which contains more than 200 calories. Plus, since beverages don't contain fiber, they won't keep you full. Stick with a smaller 8-ounce serving to minimize these liquid calories. The same goes for alcohol, which is easy to overpour. Refer to the serving size guidelines on page 265 to make sure your cocktail is a reasonable size.

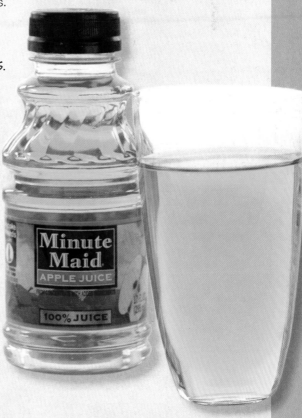

juices

Squeeze some extra nutrients into your diet with fruit and vegetable juices, but be sure to watch your portion size.

nutritional benefits

Eating fruits and vegetables helps keep you healthy and protects against disease, but it's not always easy to consume as much produce as experts advise. Fortunately, juices can be a convenient way to squeeze in extra servings. An 8-ounce glass—just 1 cup of juice—counts as one serving of a fruit or vegetable. Plus, 100% pure juices are excellent sources of vitamins and minerals, and some are enhanced with extra vitamins (such as vitamin C), minerals (such as calcium), and omega-3s. These juices may be a good idea if they're fortified with nutrients you don't get enough of in your normal diet. Make sure you buy ones labeled "100% juice" with no added sugar.

disadvantages

Juices are a concentrated source of calories, so you still need to watch how much you drink. And while they provide many of the benefits you get from eating fresh fruits and vegetables, there are some benefits that are noticeably missing. One of the key losses is fiber, which is beneficial to controlling cholesterol levels and increasing satiety. Also, when fruit is pressed to extract the juice, some antioxidants are left behind when the skins and seeds are removed. Also, vegetable juices may be high in sodium due to added salt that acts as a preservative and flavor enhancer. Look for versions with less sodium.

drinks

fyi

"from concentrate"

Juice made from concentrate is the same as the original juice. The only thing missing is most of the water. Extracting water reduces juice volume and weight, which makes it easier to ship. When water is added back to the concentrate, the product is labeled "reconstituted" or "made from concentrate" and generally has the same nutrition profile as the original juice. The exception is if sugar is added when the juice is reconstituted. Check the ingredient list to be sure.

One serving of juice has more calories and less fiber than a serving of fruit or vegetables.

juices, continued

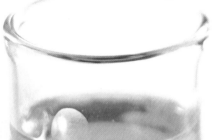

Why does juice have more calories than fruit?

To make juice, all the good-for-you fiber and solid components of the fruit (which don't contain much sugar) are removed, leaving behind a liquid that contains a higher percentage of sugar. More sugar means more calories. One serving of grapes contain 31 calories, which is just a fraction of the 116 calories found in a 6-ounce serving of grape juice.

drinks

juice drinks

"Juice drinks," "beverages," and "cocktails" may sound healthy, but they might not be the juice you think they are.

what to look for

The difference between "100% juice" and "juice drinks," "juice beverages," and "juice cocktails" is determined by the amount of juice the drink contains. Only 100% juice can be labeled "juice." Mixed juices can be labeled "100% juice" if each of the juices added to the mixture is itself 100% juice. Anything less than 100% juice must be labeled under another name. "Juice drink," "beverage," "cocktail," "punch," "blend," and "sparkler" products might contain as little as 10% or as much as 99% juice. The rest is water or added sweeteners. Check the label to find out how much juice these products contain. The ingredients must be listed on the label in the order of volume. The lower "juice" appears on the ingredient list, the less there is of it in the drink.

Some "juice drinks" may contain as little as 10% juice.

coffee

Thanks to a growing list of benefits, coffee has gone from a guilty habit to one that's good for you. But you do need to watch what you add to your morning (or afternoon) cup of joe.

nutritional benefits

At around 5 calories per 8-ounce serving, black coffee won't wreck your diet, but all the sweet additions can bulk it up to a dessert-quality treat with 300 or more calories. When fixing your coffee, keep it simple: Use a fat-free or low-fat milk in place of half-and-half (or just add a little) to get a boost of calcium, and limit how much sugar you stir in. By doing so, you keep your calories in check and still reap the nutritional benefits. Research suggests both regular and decaffeinated coffee may help protect against heart disease, Parkinson's disease, colon cancer, and type 2 diabetes.

believe it or not...

A 12-ounce whole-milk Cinnamon Dolce Latte at Starbucks® delivers nearly 300 calories; a nonfat plain has 100 calories.

How healthy is your latte?

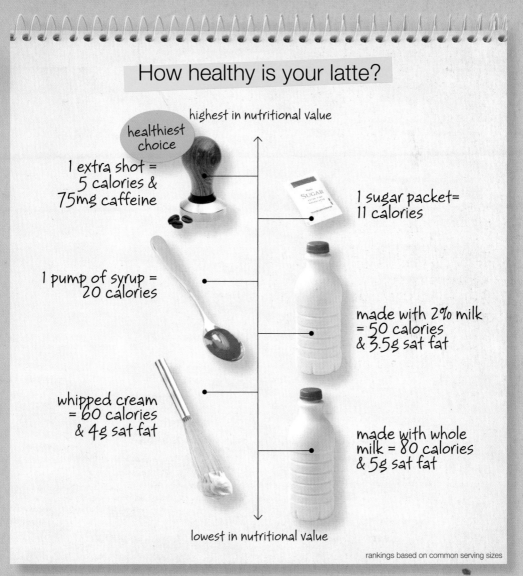

highest in nutritional value

healthiest choice

1 extra shot = 5 calories & 75mg caffeine

1 sugar packet= 11 calories

1 pump of syrup = 20 calories

made with 2% milk = 50 calories & 3.5g sat fat

whipped cream = 60 calories & 4g sat fat

made with whole milk = 80 calories & 5g sat fat

lowest in nutritional value

rankings based on common serving sizes

coffee, continued

 How much is too much caffeine?

Most experts define moderate caffeine intake as 300 milligrams or less.
Here's how that breaks down:
- Starbucks® tall coffee (12 ounces) = 375mg of caffeine
- Brewed coffee (8 ounces) = 60–180mg*
- Brewed decaf coffee (8 ounces) = 5–10mg
- Instant coffee (8 ounces) = 95mg
- Espresso (1 ounce) = 35mg
- Brewed tea (8 ounces) = 47mg
- Coca-Cola® (12 ounces) = 35mg
- Pepsi® (12 ounces) = 38mg
- Diet Coke® (12 ounces) = 47mg

*Caffeine content varies depending on brewing method, type of bean, roasting process, and ratio of water to coffee.

hot cocoa

A hot cup of rich cocoa a day can be good for you and your heart, but pay attention to the type you buy.

what to look for

Minimally processed cocoa powder contains antioxidants, specifically polyphenols, that may help reduce high blood pressure, reduce LDL (the "bad cholesterol"), or even provide potential cancer-fighting benefits. We're not talking about instant cocoa mix with added sweeteners and fillers—instead prepare your hot cocoa with unsweetened cocoa powder to reap the healthful rewards. If you prepare yours with milk, use a fat-free or low-fat variety, and keep the amount of added sugar to a minimum.

Research has shown that a cup of hot cocoa has twice the level of antioxidant activity of a 5-ounce glass of red wine.

tea

Cold or hot, tea may help protect your heart and reduce your risk of cancer.

nutritional benefits

Normal tea blends as well as green and black teas contain polyphenols and flavonoids—naturally occurring compounds that have antioxidant properties—that are believed to be the source of its health benefits. These compounds may play a role in reducing the risk of heart disease, heart attack, and stroke and lowering the risk for certain types of cancers. Plus, plain tea is very low in calories, as in, less than 3 per cup. If you like milk in your tea, use a fat-free or low-fat version. You'll also need to watch how many spoonfuls of sugar you add to your tea, whether the tea is hot or iced. A supersweet tea can transform your low-calorie beverage into a 120-calorie (or more) drink with lots of added sugar.

drinks

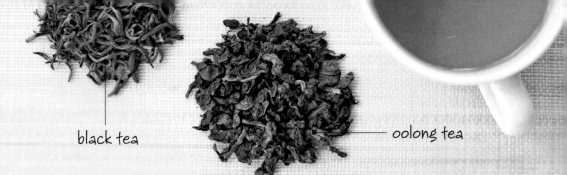

black tea

oolong tea

types of tea

fyi

Black tea, green tea, white tea, oolong tea—they all come from the *Camellia sinensis* bush but are processed differently, which is the reason for the variance in color. All are rich in antioxidants that protect you from damaging free radicals that can cause blood clots, cancer, and plaque buildup along artery walls.

white tea

green tea

Herbal tea is a blend of spices, herbs, roots, flowers, or fruit but doesn't contain tea leaves.

lemonade & flavored waters

Flavored waters can be a great alternative to plain water, but you'll need to pay attention to how many calories your favorite flavored beverage contains—it might surprise you.

what to look for

Whether you're making them yourself from a powdered mix or buying lemonade or flavored waters that are ready-made, these drinks can help you meet your daily fluid needs more easily by adding some pizzazz to plain water. And many flavored waters and powdered mixes are made with natural ingredients or artificial sweeteners that keep them calorie free or very low in calories (5 or so per serving). However, there are many on grocery store shelves that do contain calories from added sugars. For these, it's important to check the serving sizes. Even if a drink contains just 40 calories per serving, many standard 20-ounce bottles contain 2 to 2.5 servings, which can translate to a beverage with more calories than you bargained for.

Watch out for flavored waters and mixes made with sugars.

Added sugars (in the form of sugar or others like high-fructose corn syrup) in flavored waters or mixes simply mean you're taking in excess calories that don't have any nutritional value. The average mix contains 90 calories per 8-ounce serving when prepared. If you have a few glasses, you've consumed as many calories as a small meal or snack. It's fine on occasion, but if you regularly drink these beverages, you might want to consider making the switch to a brand that contains zero or very few calories per serving.

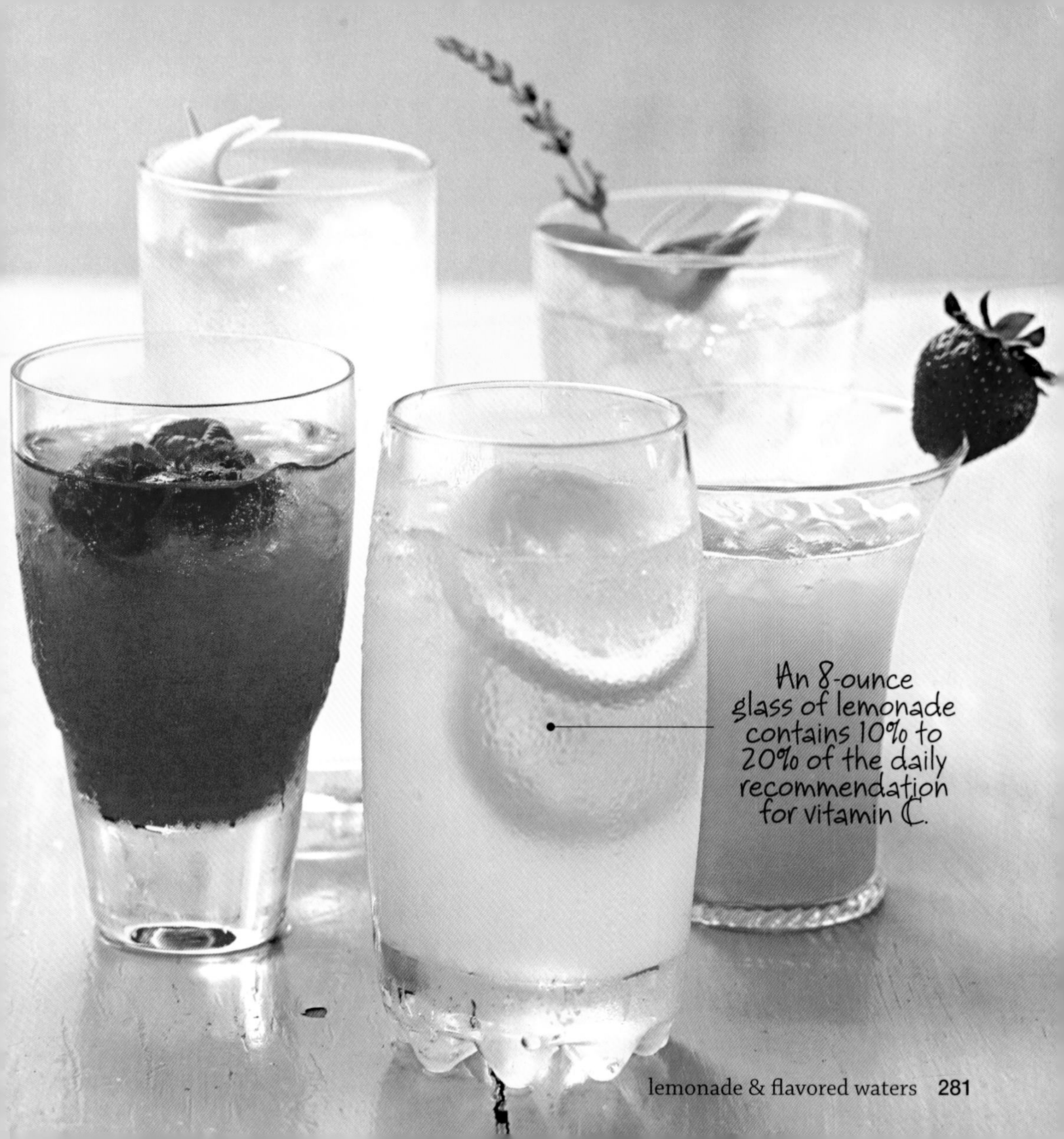

An 8-ounce
glass of lemonade
contains 10% to
20% of the daily
recommendation
for vitamin C.

sports drinks

Sports drinks offer some benefits that are great for the serious athlete, but they aren't so great for the light exerciser.

nutritional benefits

If you're engaged in light physical activity like going for a walk or doing housework, or if you exercise for less than an hour a day, skip the sports drinks. While most contain important electrolytes, such as potassium and sodium, that are necessary for intense workouts or endurance training, sports drinks are not needed to fuel light activity. Many sports drinks contain 125 calories or more per 20-ounce bottle, so spare yourself the extra calories and opt for plain water or a calorie-free beverage to keep you hydrated.

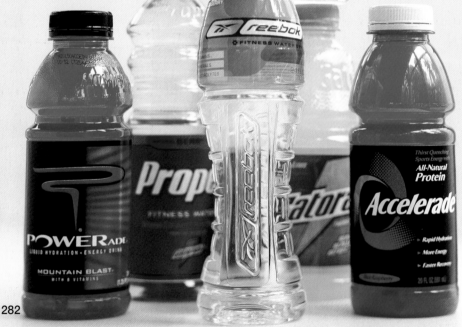

drinks

soda

Soda is certainly a popular beverage choice, but it has zero nutritional value. If you drink more than one a day, you may be taking in hundreds of extra calories.

nutrition facts

The simple truth is that sodas, both regular and diet, do not have any nutritional value whatsoever. Regular sodas are filled with added sugar (which provides lots of calories) and not much else. And although diet sodas contain few, if any, calories, they still don't contribute any vitamins, minerals, or nutrients to your diet. Plus, both contain carbolic acid through carbonation, which weakens tooth enamel, causing cavities and tooth decay. If you drink them, do so in moderation and make sure these drinks aren't replacing other more nutritious beverages like milk, juice, or water.

believe it or not...

One 21-ounce regular Coke®—the size of a medium fast-food restaurant drink—contains 210 calories and 58 grams of sugar. That's equivalent to drinking more than ¼ cup of sugar.

alcohol

Most health authorities recognize that moderate alcohol intake can be beneficial to your health. The key word is *moderate.*

nutritional benefits

Few health authorities recommend that you add alcohol to your diet if it's not something you currently enjoy, but most now recognize that moderate consumption of any alcohol—not just wine—can improve heart health. But moderation is key. Women should limit alcoholic beverages to no more than one serving daily, and for men, the limit is two (see page 265 for information about serving sizes). Any

benefit alcohol provides can be undone by drinking more than what is recommended. And if you're taking certain medications, you may need to put this habit on hold.

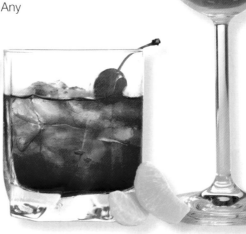
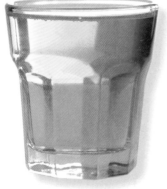

drinks

Up the nutrition ante of cocktails by adding 100% fruit juice or purees.

wine benefits

The antioxidants found in wine can vary widely depending on the year and region in which the wine was produced. However, two other beneficial components of wine remain relatively consistent: potassium, which helps maintain fluid balance in the body, and alcohol, which may help raise "good" HDL cholesterol, reduce the risk of blood clots, and lower blood pressure. The key to obtaining wine's benefits is enjoying your favorite in moderation—no more than one and two glasses per day for women and men, respectively.

refrigerated & frozen foods

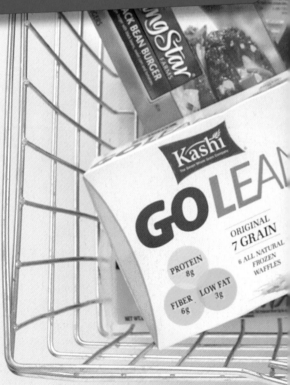

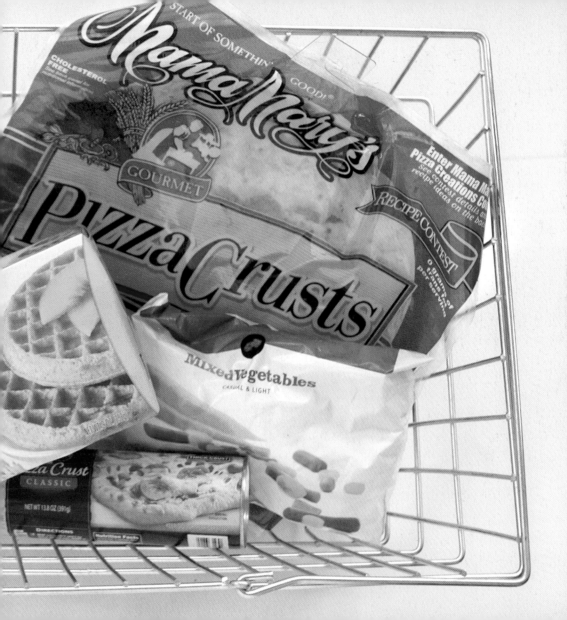

refrigerated & frozen foods

Why eat refrigerated and frozen foods?

The healthiest refrigerated and frozen foods can be a source of:

- ☑ fruits and vegetables
- ☑ high-quality protein
- ☑ whole grains and fiber
- ☑ healthy unsaturated fats
- ☑ few, if any, saturated fats

How much should I eat?

The serving sizes for these foods vary. For frozen produce, see the guidelines on page 30. For biscuits, rolls, cinnamon rolls, and doughs, use the guidelines on page 66. For pastas, refer to page 190. Tofu, tempeh, and vegetable burgers can help you meet your daily protein needs of about 30 to 45 grams. See page 110 for more information. Plus, throughout this chapter, we give guidelines on proper portions to help you.

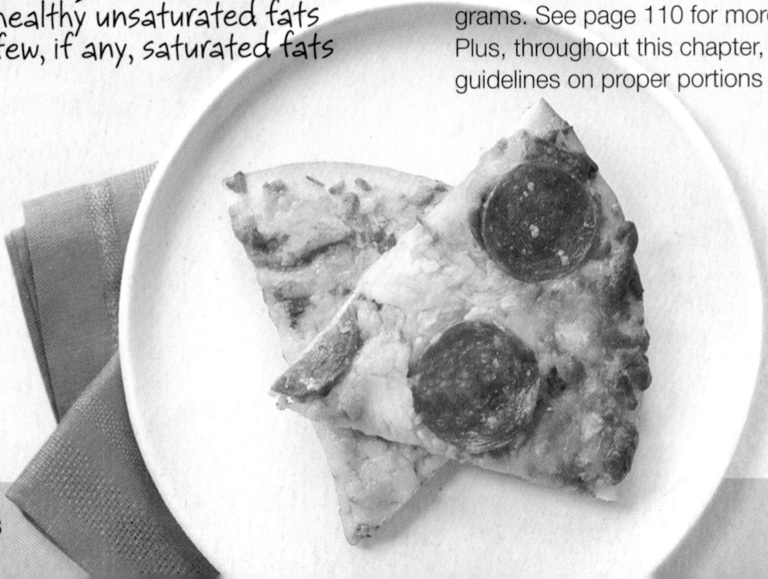

What is a serving?

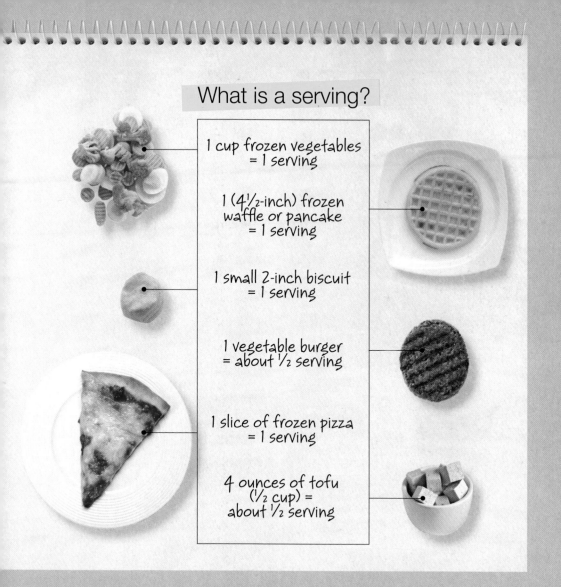

1 cup frozen vegetables
= 1 serving

1 (4½-inch) frozen
waffle or pancake
= 1 serving

1 small 2-inch biscuit
= 1 serving

1 vegetable burger
= about ½ serving

1 slice of frozen pizza
= 1 serving

4 ounces of tofu
(½ cup) =
about ½ serving

choose the <mark>healthiest</mark> refrigerated & frozen foods

The refrigerated and frozen foods aisles offer a variety of healthy options if you know what to look for.

1. Keep it simple.

In these sections, simple foods can be key. In general, the healthiest choices are those that haven't been overly prepared by the manufacturer. For example, frozen vegetables that include just vegetables (one or a mix) are generally a healthier choice than packages that include vegetables covered in salty seasonings and cheesy sauces. We show you what to look for on the following pages.

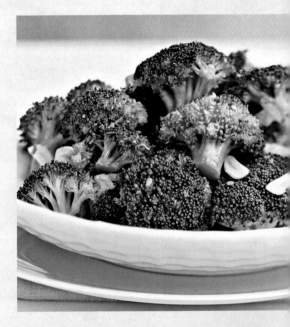

2. Look for foods that are healthier versions of themselves.

Food manufacturers have produced healthier versions of many food products, including refrigerated and frozen foods. Look for those when shopping. You'll find healthy produce, whole grains, and leaner sources of protein, plus healthy additions (think flax, wheat germ, added fruits and vegetables) that amp up the nutritional package of some convenient and easy refrigerator and freezer favorites.

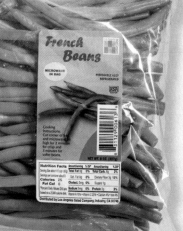

3. Keep portion size in mind.

Refrigerated and frozen foods can be calorically dense, so a small portion size might contain way more calories (and saturated fat and sodium) than you think. Read nutrition labels carefully so you know what you're buying before you bring it home.

watch out for these red flags

The refrigerated and frozen foods sections offer a bevy of convenient food options, but these products can be some of the worst nutritional offenders in the grocery store.

Watch out for saturated fat, trans fats, and sodium.

In some cases, convenience comes at a high nutritional cost, since many of these foods are filled with saturated fat, trans fat, and sodium. Some products carry more than a day's worth of each of these in one serving. Read the nutrition labels and ingredient lists closely to make sure the products you're buying aren't a nutritional nightmare. And follow our guidelines throughout the chapter to help you navigate these aisles effectively.

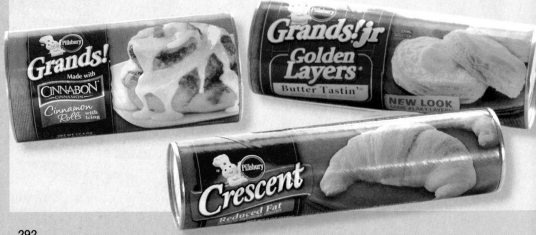

⚑ Watch out for serving sizes.

The serving sizes for some of these products may surprise you. You may think the individual meal you're eating is just one serving, but the manufacturer may consider it to be two. Check the serving size on the label to make sure you're not taking in double (or triple) what you think you are.

⚑ Watch out for higher cost.

Convenience carries a higher price tag, since much of the work is done for you. And because many of the items in the refrigerated and frozen aisles are premade and prepackaged, you can expect to pay more.

> Convenience products carry a higher price tag, since part of the work is done for you.

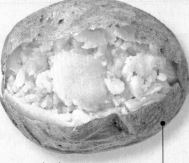

baking potatoes: $0.99 per pound.

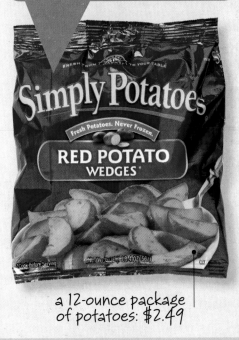

a 12-ounce package of potatoes: $2.49

293

tofu & tempeh

Both tofu and tempeh are made from soy, which offers a lean source of protein with minimal saturated fat and sodium.

what to look for

The soy protein in tofu and tempeh may help reduce the risk of heart disease. Plus, these items are both low in saturated fat and sodium.

tofu

Tofu is low in calories—3 ounces generally contains 30 to 65 calories—and it's a storehouse of vitamins and minerals, including folic acid and iron. It comes in a variety of textures—from silken to extra firm. Nutritionally, there's not a lot of difference from variations in texture, but you can save calories (up to 39%) by choosing light tofu over regular tofu.

tempeh

Tempeh contains more calories than tofu—a 3-ounce serving contains 110 to 165 calories—but it also contains more protein. It can be made from just soybeans, but you'll often find the soy mixed with a grain, such as rice, barley, or quinoa. All-soy tempeh is the highest in protein, but it's also the highest in fat. But any variety of tempeh is a healthy choice, so choose one that offers the best flavor.

Just ⅓ cup of tofu made with calcium sulfate has about 30% of the daily recommendation for calcium.

tofu and calcium

Tofu can also be a great nondairy source of calcium. But make sure you choose a brand that's made with calcium sulfate—one 3-ounce portion (⅛ cup) contains 300 milligrams of calcium. Nigari (magnesium chloride) is another common coagulating agent used to make tofu, but its calcium content is lower—3 ounces may contain as little as 20 milligrams of calcium.

Q&A What's the difference between tofu and tempeh?

Both tofu and tempeh are made from soy. Tofu is made by coagulating soy milk and then pressing it into blocks. Tempeh is made by fermenting soybeans with a mold that's then pressed into patties.

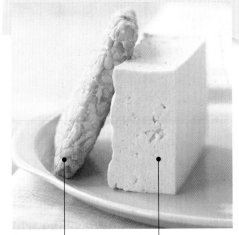

A 3-ounce piece of tempeh contains around 18 grams of protein.

A 3-ounce piece of tofu contains around 6 grams of protein.

refrigerated pasta

When buying pasta, you don't have to limit yourself to the dry varieties. Many grocery stores carry fresh pasta in the refrigerated sections.

what to look for

One of the healthiest choices among fresh pasta is the 100% whole-wheat variety. Made with whole-wheat flour, this type counts towards the recommended three servings of whole grains you need per day; plus, it provides a healthy dose of fiber. Stuffed pastas that contain cheese, such as ravioli and tortellini, are generally higher in fat and calories. For these pastas, look for a light variety that is lower in calories, saturated fat, and sodium.

Watch out for sodium.

Read the labels carefully to compare the whole-wheat variety to regular fresh pastas. Some brands of whole-wheat pasta may be higher in sodium than traditional pasta.

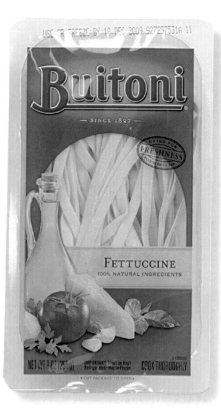

pizza dough

Refrigerated pizza dough—in its many forms—can be a great base to a healthy meal.

what to look for

From thin crust to classic, there are several different types of refrigerated pizza crusts for you to try. Ideally, you should choose a product that is 100% whole wheat, but those can sometimes be more difficult to find. Many pizza doughs have similar calorie levels per serving, but you might notice differences in fat (particularly saturated fat) and sodium among them. Read the labels carefully, and choose one that has 1.5 grams of saturated fat or less per serving and the least amount of sodium. And if you're watching your calories closely, go with thin crust over regular or thick—it has less calories per slice.

fyi whole-wheat crust

Nutritionally, whole-wheat crusts have their competition beat. One slice (a sixth of a 10-ounce thin crust) packs in more than 4 grams of fiber. The regular crusts don't even provide 1 gram for a similarly sized slice.

pizza dough, continued

types of crusts

There are several varieties available for you to choose from.

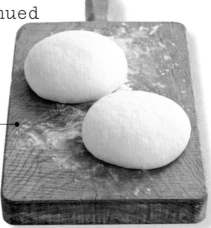

fresh pizza dough

Some grocery stores make their own pizza dough every day. Check to see if your store carries a whole-wheat variety.

One-sixth of an 11-ounce crust: 137 calories, 1.4g fat (0g sat fat), 319mg sodium

prebaked pizza crust

The premade packaged pizza crusts are generally the most expensive pizza crust options in the grocery store.

One-sixth of a 12-inch crust: 179 calories, 5.8g fat (1g sat fat), 185mg sodium

refrigerated pizza dough

These tubes of crusts are easy to use and easy to find.

One-sixth of a 13.8-ounce regular crust: 174 calories, 3.5g fat (1.2g sat fat), 348mg sodium

One-sixth of a 10-ounce thin crust: 141 calories, 2.9g fat (1.2g sat fat), 274mg sodium

One-sixth of a 10-ounce whole-wheat thin crust: 124 calories, 2.5g fat (1.2g sat fat), 232mg sodium

By making your own pizza at home instead of ordering in, you can save some cash and also take in fewer calories—about 15% less per slice.

pizza dough, continued

five smart topping trade-offs

We did the nutritional math to calculate simple switches that add up to big calorie, fat, and sodium savings. With our picks, you can have your pie and eat it too.

tomato-based sauce

This option has about half the sodium of a white sauce counterpart (made of eggs, cream, and some-times cheese), plus going red helps you avoid 8 grams of saturated fat.

chicken apple sausage

While it's not surprising that poultry is a healthier choice than Italian pork sausage, it is shocking that the poultry version has half the calories, fat, and saturated fat, compared to the same portion of pork.

refrigerated & frozen foods

Spanish chorizo

For cured meat, super-seasoned chorizo beats pepperoni with 20 fewer calories and 80 fewer milligrams of sodium in similar serving sizes.

kalamata olives

They deliver the same briny, salty notes of anchovies, but olives make a better choice because a comparable portion undercuts anchovies' sodium level by half.

bacon

It has all the savory, porky notes of pancetta (and a comparable amount of saturated fat), but it contains half the sodium of the Italian version.

canned biscuits & dinner rolls

When you need something easy to round out a meal, refrigerated biscuits and rolls may be your go-to option. Here are a few things to keep in mind.

what to look for

Refrigerated biscuits and rolls are quick and convenient, but some can pack a lot of calories and saturated fat into that tiny tube of dough. Go for whole-wheat varieties when available to get in some fiber and whole grains. Reduced-fat varieties provide a small amount of calorie savings, but the real benefit is the reduction of saturated fat—about 1 gram per biscuit. Whatever type you buy, look for one that has around 130 calories or less, the least amount of saturated fat as possible (preferably 3 grams or less), and 350 milligrams of sodium or less per biscuit or roll.

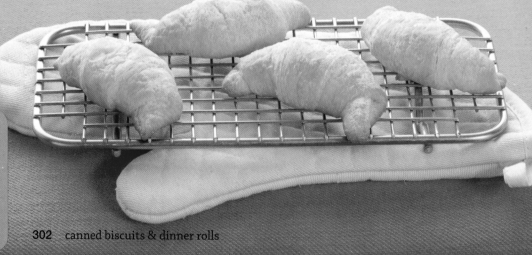

It probably won't come as a surprise that store-bought biscuits are *much* better for you than those found in the drive-through lane, but you might not realize how much better. The average store-bought biscuit has 110 calories, 1.5 grams of saturated fat, and 350 milligrams of sodium. A regular-sized biscuit at a fast-food restaurant has 260 calories, 7 grams of saturated fat, and 740 milligrams of sodium *per biscuit.*

Watch out for "wheat."

The term "wheat" on the package doesn't necessarily mean it's a better choice nutritionally. Often these products are made with refined wheat flour, which doesn't offer many benefits, since most of the nutrition has been stripped out. Plus, in addition to not being better for you, these healthier-sounding "wheat" biscuits or rolls can carry a load of calories per serving—as much as 200 calories each. The key words are "whole wheat," which means it's a whole grain. Look for it on the package or near the beginning on the ingredient list. (See page 69 for more information about identifying whole grains.)

canned cinnamon rolls

The blend of soft dough made with refined flour and icing is certainly delicious, but nutritionally, the mix isn't so sweet.

what to look for

Cinnamon rolls are a treat that's definitely sweet, but there's really nothing healthy about them at all. They're calorie-dense and contain saturated fats and usually trans fats—sometimes more than two days' worth in one roll. It's best to save these for an occasional splurge and enjoy them in moderation. If you eat cinnamon rolls more regularly, consider downsizing from the extra-large rolls to the smaller ones and then from the smaller ones to the reduced-fat variety. And then don't go back for seconds at the breakfast table.

refrigerated & frozen foods

calorie comparison

Here's the nutritional breakdown for some common canned cinnamon rolls:

Pillsbury® Grands Cinnamon Rolls (1 roll):
370 calories
5g sat fat
5g trans fat

Pillsbury® Cinnamon Rolls (1 roll):
140 calories
1.5g sat fat
2g trans fat

Pillsbury® Reduced-Fat Cinnamon Rolls (1 roll):
130 calories
2.5g sat fat
0g trans fat

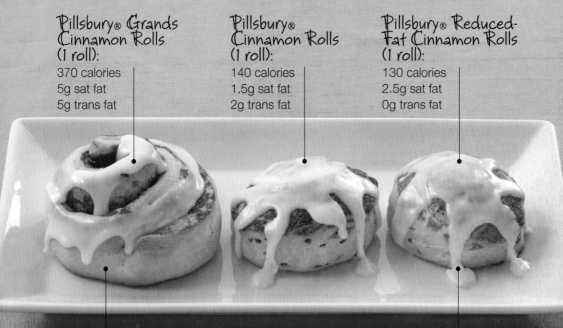

This roll contains more than a days' worth of the recommended maximum amount of trans fats in one roll.

This nutrition label says 0 grams of trans fats, but this roll has partially hydrogenated oil listed as one of the ingredients, so it's not really trans fat free.

refrigerated & frozen potatoes

Potatoes are popular and come in many forms that can be served for breakfast, lunch, and dinner.

what to look for

Mashed, sliced, diced, or fried, you're sure to find one of these potato versions in the refrigerated or freezer sections. And once there, you'll notice some good things and some not-so-good things. Many convenient potato products are fried before being refrigerated or frozen, and some use partially hydrogenated oils. The healthiest options have potatoes listed first in the ingredient list. They also use vegetable or canola oil—not partially hydrogenated oil—which means the saturated fat content should be low (preferably less than 1 gram per serving) and they'll be trans fat free. Be aware that sodium levels can be very high in these products, especially the seasoned varieties. Choose one that has no more that 300 milligrams of sodium per serving.

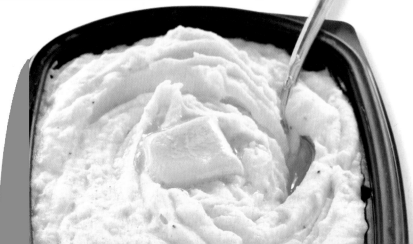

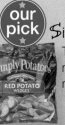
Sweet potato fries are a great choice. One 3-ounce serving (less than what's shown below) contains 100% of the daily recommendation for vitamin A and 10% for vitamin C.

frozen fruits & vegetables

Frozen fruits and vegetables can be just as healthy as their fresh counterparts, and they can help get you through the off-season when your favorite fresh fruits and vegetables aren't at their best.

what to look for

Frozen fruits and vegetables are just as healthy for you as fresh, since they have been frozen at the peak of freshness and nutrition. Plus, when fruits and vegetables are out of season, the frozen version can often be cheaper than the fresh ones flown in from warmer locales.

Watch out for added salt or sugar.
When shopping for frozen fruits and vegetables, check the ingredient list. Some varieties include added salt and sugar that you don't need. (See page 237 for more information about identifying added sugars.) Instead, choose ones that only contain the vegetable or fruit you're looking for.

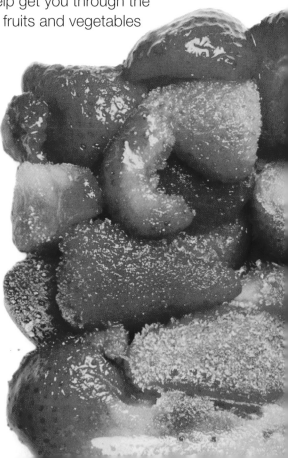

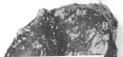

frozen waffles & pancakes

These quick and convenient breakfast options can be healthy choices depending on the type you buy and all of the sweet condiments you add to them.

what to look for

Many frozen waffles and pancakes are high in fat and full of added sugar, but there are some healthy options out there. Look for products that include whole-wheat flour, bran, whole grains, natural or organic ingredients, and minimal added sugars. Ideally, one frozen waffle or pancake will contain 90 calories or less, zero grams of saturated and trans fats, 1 gram of fiber or more, and 5 grams of sugar or less. Some waffle varieties also have added benefits like flax seeds, which are rich in omega-3 fats and may help lower cholesterol.

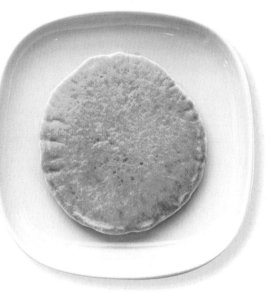

Watch out for added sugar.
Avoid products with sugary sweet ingredients like chocolate chips. They're fine for a once-in-a-while treat, but all that sugar isn't ideal for an everyday meal.

Watch out for the condiments you add.

The average syrup contains a hefty 210 calories and 32 grams of sugar in just ¼ cup. Our advice: Use less of the regular variety or switch to a "lite" syrup that contains half of the calories of regular. An even better substitution would be to swap the syrup for fresh berries or bananas. See more information about syrup on page 170.

frozen biscuits & breakfast sandwiches

Some people can't get enough of these easy breakfast options. It's too bad they're not better for you.

what to look for

Frozen biscuits and breakfast sandwiches

While most frozen biscuits and breakfast sandwiches in the freezer section are high in unhealthy saturated fat and trans fat and carry a load of excess calories, you can find a few healthier choices. Look for brands that use lean turkey sausage, egg whites, and whole-grain breads (or a bread made with whole grains)—preferably one that has less than 300 calories, 4 grams of saturated fat or less, 0 grams of trans fat, and at least 2 grams of fiber.

Frozen sausage

A two-patty serving of a typical pork breakfast sausage will leave you with 8 grams of saturated fat when you get up from the breakfast table—that's more than half of the daily recommendation. A healthier option is turkey sausage, which has an average of 120 calories and 2 grams of saturated fat in a two-patty serving. All sausages are usually high in sodium, so be sure to compare labels and choose the one that contains the least amount per serving.

believe it or not...

A regular bacon, egg, and cheese biscuit from a popular drive-through contains more than 400 calories, 12 grams of saturated fat (more than 75% of the daily recommendation), and almost 1,200 milligrams of sodium (more than half the recommended amount per day). That certainly isn't the best way to start the day.

This frozen breakfast sandwich is a healthier choice when compared to drive-through options. It contains lean turkey sausage, egg whites, and bread made with whole grains. However, it's still high in sodium: 760 milligrams for one sandwich. Keep that in mind.

frozen pizza

Frozen pizzas put a quick dinner within easy reach, but options that are both tasty and nutritious are sometimes hard to come by.

what to look for

Finding healthy frozen pizzas that also taste delicious can be a challenge. Thin-crust pizzas are generally lower in calories, since the crust is noticeably thinner than regular and thick-crust pizzas. Look for brands that contain 350 calories or less, 6 grams or less of saturated fat, and a reasonable amount of sodium (400 milligrams or less) per slice. Also, be sure to check the ingredient list and choose one that doesn't contain partially hydrogenated oils—you don't need those trans fats.

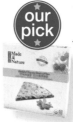

our pick

Made in Nature® Organic Gourmet Three Cheese Pizza

The thick crust and melty cheese made this one a winner.

our pick

Whole Foods® 365 Chicken Caesar Pizza

We liked the crispy crust and Caesar flavor profile.

believe it or not...

At the rate Americans eat pizza, you'd think it was an official food guide pyramid category. The amount of pizza we consume in a day is best measured in acres—100 to be exact. (That's about the size of 100 football fields.) And given how pizza can quickly turn into a nutritional nightmare, it's no wonder we have an obesity crisis. Two slices of a certain purveyor's large Italian sausage and red onion pizza tally up to 700 calories and 1,720 milligrams of sodium.

refrigerated & frozen foods

Made in Nature® Organic Gourmet Three Cheese Pizza

Whole Foods® 365 Chicken Caesar Pizza

frozen vegetable burgers

Done right, vegetable burgers are full of delicious flavors and are packed with nutrition, courtesy of lean vegetable protein and fiber.

nutritional benefits

Frozen vegetable burgers offer a great way to keep your saturated fat intake in check. Even though soy-based burgers and vegetable burgers are naturally cholesterol free and have similar calorie and fiber profiles, soy provides more protein and about four times more iron and calcium. But both options are healthy, so choose the one you like best.

our pick Sunshine® Southwest Organic Burger

This hefty burger has big flavor courtesy of cumin and jalapeño pepper, but it still manages a low sodium count. Plus, it has plenty of healthy fiber. Spread fat-free refried beans on the bun to boost protein. For extra nutrition credit, top with a tablespoon or two of guacamole. ————————

our pick Morningstar Farms® Spicy Black Bean Burger

Besides good amounts of satiating fiber and protein, this patty boasts a trim calorie count. That means you can add a hearty 100% whole-grain bun, half an ounce of Monterey Jack cheese, lettuce, and tomato, plus a tasty spread. ————————

our pick Amy's® California Veggie Burger ————————

Balanced taste and texture make Amy's stand out among other options. Like the Sunshine burger, this patty's protein is on the low end. To increase it, add an ounce of extra-sharp, reduced-fat Cheddar cheese; try it with a whole-wheat baguette and fixings.

frozen entrées

Whether you want to lose or maintain a healthy weight or simply don't feel like preparing a meal, packaged frozen entrées can be a convenient and healthy portion-controlled option.

what to look for

From low-calorie and organic to ethnic and vegetarian, there is a wide variety of convenient frozen entrées available. Some are healthy, while others are not so healthy. Read the ingredient list: The best meals are those that list healthy, natural ingredients first. Look for vegetables, beans, whole grains like brown rice, and lean meats like fish and poultry. Also, look for meals that contain a moderate amount of calories (500 or less), have at least 5 grams of fiber, are low in saturated fat (4 grams or less), and contain less than 600 milligrams of sodium per serving. And perhaps most importantly, check the serving size. Some individually portioned meals contain more than one serving, and some don't provide enough calories to be a full meal (see "portion control" box on page 319).

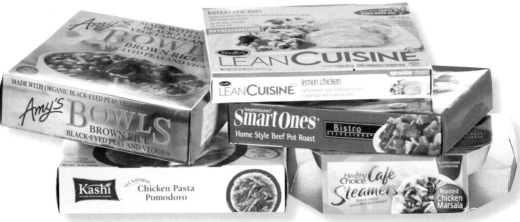

refrigerated & frozen foods

Watch out for sodium.

Many frozen meals, including the "healthy" ones, are loaded with salt—some have close to 2,000 milligrams of sodium per serving. Be sure to check the nutrition label to make sure the sodium amount is reasonable (less than 600 milligrams per serving). You can also look for frozen meals that are labeled "reduced sodium" or "heart healthy," although not all lower-sodium options will be labeled this way.

fyi portion control

Frozen individual meals are a great way to help you practice portion control, since the amount is set and you aren't tempted to go back for seconds. However, some aren't hefty enough to be a full meal. Those that are less than 400 calories usually need to be supplemented with a healthy side, like fresh fruit or a salad.

frozen family dinners

Walk down the freezer aisle in your grocery store, and it's easy to see that frozen dinners are popular and aren't lacking in variety. What they're often lacking in, though, is nutrition.

what to look for

While they're convenient, frozen family-size dinners don't have many redeeming nutritional qualities. Most are packed with calories, saturated fat, and sodium. Plus, based on the serving sizes, some frozen dinners serve as many as 12 people—more servings than many consumers realize. Unfortunately, there aren't many "good-for-you" options available. Resort to these only once in a while, and be sure to check the label to see how many servings one dinner is supposed to serve so you know what you're buying.

Watch out for serving sizes. If one family-size dinner is a meal for your family of four, then you might want to take a closer look at the nutrition label and see how many servings that convenient dinner contains. The widely available brand shown on page 321 contains 12 servings—one serving contains 340 calories, 7 grams of saturated fat (about half of the daily recommended amount) and 650 milligrams of sodium (more than a quarter of the daily recommendation). So, if you're having more than one serving, you're taking in a lot of unhealthy extras that aren't doing your waistline—or your heart—any favors.

This dish may be easy and convenient, but it's also loaded with calories, saturated fat, and sodium.

metric equivalents

The information in the following charts is provided to help cooks outside the United States successfully convert measurements mentioned in this book. All equivalents are approximate.

Equivalents for Different Types of Ingredients

Standard Cup	Fine Powder (ex. flour)	Grain (ex. rice)	Granular (ex. sugar)	Liquid Solids (ex. butter)	Liquid (ex. milk)
1	140 g	150 g	190 g	200 g	240 ml
¾	105 g	113 g	143 g	150 g	180 ml
⅔	93 g	100 g	125 g	133 g	160 ml
½	70 g	75 g	95 g	100 g	120 ml
⅓	47 g	50 g	63 g	67 g	80 ml
¼	35 g	38 g	48 g	50 g	60 ml
⅛	18 g	19 g	24 g	25 g	30 ml

Liquid Ingredients by Volume

¼ tsp			=	1 ml
½ tsp			=	2 ml
1 tsp			=	5 ml
3 tsp =	1 tbl	= ½ fl oz =		15 ml
	2 tbls = ⅛ cup	= 1 fl oz =		30 ml
	4 tbls = ¼ cup	= 2 fl oz =		60 ml
	5⅓ tbls = ⅓ cup	= 3 fl oz =		80 ml
	8 tbls = ½ cup	= 4 fl oz =		120 ml
	10⅔ tbls = ⅔ cup	= 5 fl oz =		160 ml
	12 tbls = ¾ cup	= 6 fl oz =		180 ml
	16 tbls = 1 cup	= 8 fl oz =		240 ml
	1 pt = 2 cups = 16 fl oz =			480 ml
	1 qt = 4 cups = 32 fl oz =			960 ml
	33 fl oz = 1000 ml = 1 l			

Length
(To convert inches to centimeters, multiply the number of inches by 2.5.)

1 in =		2.5 cm
6 in = ½ ft		= 15 cm
12 in = 1 ft		= 30 cm
36 in = 3 ft = 1 yd		= 90 cm
40 in =		100 cm = 1 m

Dry Ingredients by Weight
(To convert ounces to grams, multiply the number of ounces by 30.)

1 oz	=	¹⁄₁₆ lb	=	30 g
4 oz	=	¼ lb	=	120 g
8 oz	=	½ lb	=	240 g
12 oz	=	¾ lb	=	360 g
16 oz	=	1 lb	=	480 g

Cooking/Oven Temperatures

	Fahrenheit	Celsius	Gas Mark
Freeze Water	32° F	0° C	
Room Temp.	68° F	20° C	
Boil Water	212° F	100° C	
Bake	325° F	160° C	3
	350° F	180° C	4
	375° F	190° C	5
	400° F	200° C	6
	425° F	220° C	7
	450° F	230° C	8
Broil			Grill

nutritional guide

Daily Nutrition Guide

These guidelines are a daily reference guide and supplement the recommendations throughout this book. Remember that one size does not fit all. Take lifestyle, age, and circumstances into consideration. For example, pregnant or breast-feeding women need more protein, calories, and calcium. Those who are less active need fewer calories and protein. Go to mypyramid.gov for your own personalized plan.

	Women ages 25 to 50	Women over 50	Men over 24
Calories	2,000	2,000 or less	2,700
Protein	50g	50g or less	63g
Fat	65g or less	65g or less	88g or less
Saturated Fat	20g or less	20g or less	27g or less
Carbohydrates	304g	304g	410g
Fiber	25g to 35g	25g to 35g	25g to 35g
Cholesterol	300mg or less	300mg or less	300mg or less
Iron	18mg	8mg	8mg
Sodium	2,300mg or less	1,500mg or less	2,300mg or less
Calcium	1,000mg	1,200mg	1,000mg

These nutrition guidelines are general recommendations for individuals who get more than 30 minutes per day of moderate physical activity beyond normal activities.

glossary of nutrition terms

Amino acids: Organic molecules that are the building blocks of proteins.

Anthocyanin (an-THO-cyan-in): Part of the flavonoid family of compounds, this blue-tinted antioxidant may bolster memory and healthy aging.

Antioxidants: A family of chemicals, such as carotenoids and vitamins C and E, found naturally in plants. They help neutralize free radicals and keep cells healthy.

Carotenoid (kur-OT-en-oid): A family of phytonutrients; vibrantly colored pigments found in fruits and vegetables, one form of which is the body's precursor to vitamin A.

Cholesterol: This compound is a vital structural component of cell membranes and helps create hormones. Dietary sources of cholesterol come from animal sources, but it's also synthesized in the liver. In atherosclerosis, cholesterol accumulates as plaque along the walls of arteries.

Ellagitannin (EL-a-gu-tan-en): An antioxidant found in berries, grapes, and kiwis; a member of the phenol class of phytonutrients.

Fat-soluble vitamins: These vitamins, which include vitamins A, D, E, and K, dissolve in fat before they are absorbed into the bloodstream. The body stores any excesses of these vitamins in the liver and fatty tissues, so they're not needed every day. Foods that contain these vitamins will not lose them when cooked.

Fiber: Besides ensuring a healthy digestive tract, fiber from foods can help you lose weight, lower blood pressure and cholesterol levels, and reduce the risk for diabetes and heart disease.

Flavonoid (FLAV-o-noid): A class of phytochemicals likely to maintain immune health and heart health and support brain function.

Free radicals: Chemicals that our body produces when cells burn oxygen for fuel during metabolism. They're unstable and attack and damage healthy cells, promoting cancer, artery damage, and heart disease.

Indoles (IN-doles): Bioactive compounds found in green and white produce that may reduce certain cancer risks.

Isoflavones: These natural chemicals are a class of phytoestrogens believed to have disease-fighting effects and are found mainly in soy foods. They also act as antioxidants.

Isothiocyanates (I-so-THI-o-cyan-ates): A class of phytonutrients found in cruciferous vegetables that may reduce cancer risks.

Lignans: Lignans are a group of chemical compounds found in plants—flaxseed and sesame seeds are rich sources. They're a class of phytoestrogens and also act as antioxidants.

Lutein (LOO-teen): A carotenoid that likely protects the eyes, reduces damage caused by free radicals, and combats cataracts.

Lycopene: A phytochemical associated with the red pigment in tomatoes, pink grapefruit, and watermelons. It's been found to have antioxidant properties that are believed to reduce the risk for cancer, heart disease, and macular degeneration.

Omega-3 fatty acids: These healthful polyunsaturated fats help improve cardiovascular health by controlling cholesterol and reducing blood pressure.

Phytochemicals/phytonutrients: Compounds that are found in all plant-based foods, including fruits, vegetables, nuts, and grains. Believed to aid in the prevention of cancer and heart disease.

Phytoestrogens: Phytoestrogens are a group of natural plant compounds that are similar, at the molecular level, to the hormone estrogen. They're believed to have a protective effect against a variety of cancers, heart disease, brain disorders, and osteoporosis.

Polyphenols: These chemical substances are found in plants and have antioxidant properties that may help reduce the risk of heart disease and cancer.

Proanthocyanidin (PRO-an-tho-cyan-i-din): This compound, in the flavonoid group of phytochemicals, likely promotes heart health.

Probiotics: These live microorganisms are added to certain foods, such as yogurt, and are believed to help stimulate the growth of good bacteria in the gastrointestinal tract when eaten in adequate amounts.

Water-soluble vitamins: These vitamins, which include B-complex vitamins and vitamin C, dissolve in water before being absorbed into the bloodstream. These must be replaced each day, since the body uses only what it needs and excretes the rest. Water-soluble vitamins are easily destroyed or washed out when foods are cooked.

Zeaxanthin (zee-uh-ZAN-thin): A carotenoid that likely supports eye health.

glossary of vitamins & minerals

Biotin: Biotin is an essential water-soluble B-complex vitamin that helps break down carbohydrates and fats.

Calcium: Calcium is the most abundant mineral in the body. Besides maintaining strong bones and teeth, it's important for muscle contraction, blood vessel expansion and contraction, hormone balance, and nerve conductivity.

Chromium: This essential mineral plays a role in carbohydrate metabolism and the maintenance of blood sugar levels.

Copper: A normal component of blood, it's also part of many enzymes, which are involved in energy production, the formation of connective tissue, and the metabolism of iron. And it plays a role in the normal function of the brain and nervous system.

Fluoride: A natural element found in nearly all drinking waters (although water purification systems filter it out), fluoride helps protect tooth enamel and prevent tooth decay. However, it's not considered an essential mineral because humans don't require it for growth or to sustain life.

Folate (folic acid): This water-soluble B-complex vitamin plays a starring role in the creation of DNA, which is why it's vital for pregnant women to get enough of it. It also helps the body make red blood cells.

Iodine: Iodine is required by humans for the creation of thyroid hormones, which play a role in proper growth, development, metabolism, and reproduction.

Iron: The majority of this mineral is found in hemoglobin, a protein in red blood cells that carries oxygen to cells and tissues. Iron is also part of myoglobin, which carries oxygen to muscles. A deficiency can leave you tired and weak.

Magnesium: Magnesium plays an important role in hundreds of body processes, including muscle and nerve function, regulation of metabolism, heart rate, blood pressure, and bone health (50% of body magnesium is found in bone).

Manganese: A component of many enzymes, it can also activate other enzymes. It's associated with the formation of connective and skeletal tissue, healthy growth and development, and the metabolism of carbohydrates and fat.

Niacin: Formerly called vitamin B_3, niacin helps the body convert food into energy. It also plays a role in nerve function and helps maintain healthy skin.

Pantothenic Acid: Formerly known as vitamin B_5, pantothenic acid is found in cells in the form of coenzyme A and is a vital part of numerous chemical reactions that sustain life, such as helping generate energy from food and helping create essential hormones.

Phosphorus: This mineral helps form healthy bones and teeth. It's part of every cell in the body and is necessary for the body to function normally.

Potassium: Potassium helps maintain your heartbeat and other muscle and nervous system functions. It, along with sodium, helps the body maintain a proper level of water in the blood and tissues.

Riboflavin: Formerly called vitamin B_2, riboflavin is vital for turning carbohydrates into energy. It's also a key component in red blood cell formation and vision.

Selenium: This trace element is essential for the proper function of some enzymes that form proteins.

Sodium (sodium chloride): Sodium (salt) is essential for life. It, along with potassium, helps keep the water content of the body properly balanced. Only a minimal amount of salt is required for survival, and the health implications of excess salt intake are a major concern.

Thiamin: Formerly called vitamin B_1, thiamin helps the body convert carbohydrates into energy. It's also vital for the heart, nervous system, and muscles to function properly.

Vitamin A: This fat-soluble vitamin is essential for the normal growth, development, and maintenance of tissues. It's essential to night vision and helps in the normal growth of bones and teeth. It also functions as an antioxidant. However, it's toxic in large doses.

Vitamin B_6: Vitamin B_6 helps your brain and nerves function properly. Plus, it helps the body make red blood cells and break down proteins.

Vitamin B_{12}: This vitamin helps make red blood cells and helps keep nerve cells functioning properly.

Vitamin C: Also called ascorbic acid, vitamin C is needed to form collagen and is essential for healthy bones, teeth, gums, and blood vessels. It also assists in wound healing, and it helps the body absorb calcium and iron.

Vitamin D: This fat-soluble vitamin keeps bones and teeth healthy by helping the body absorb calcium. It's also unique because the body can manufacture it when skin is exposed to sunlight.

Vitamin E: The main job of this fat-soluble vitamin is that of an antioxidant—it protects the body from damage caused by free radicals. It also helps keep red blood cells healthy.

Vitamin K: This fat-soluble vitamin is essential for blood clotting.

Zinc: This mineral plays an important role in wound healing, growth, and the maintenance of a healthy immune system.

index